Books may be purchased by contacting the publisher at:
www.enhancetheuk.org

Cover design: Jamie Bartlett

First Edition, 2015

ISBN 978-0-9934242-1-2

✦ enhance the uk
changing society's views on disability

Undressing Disability
by Enhance The UK

Contents

Introduction

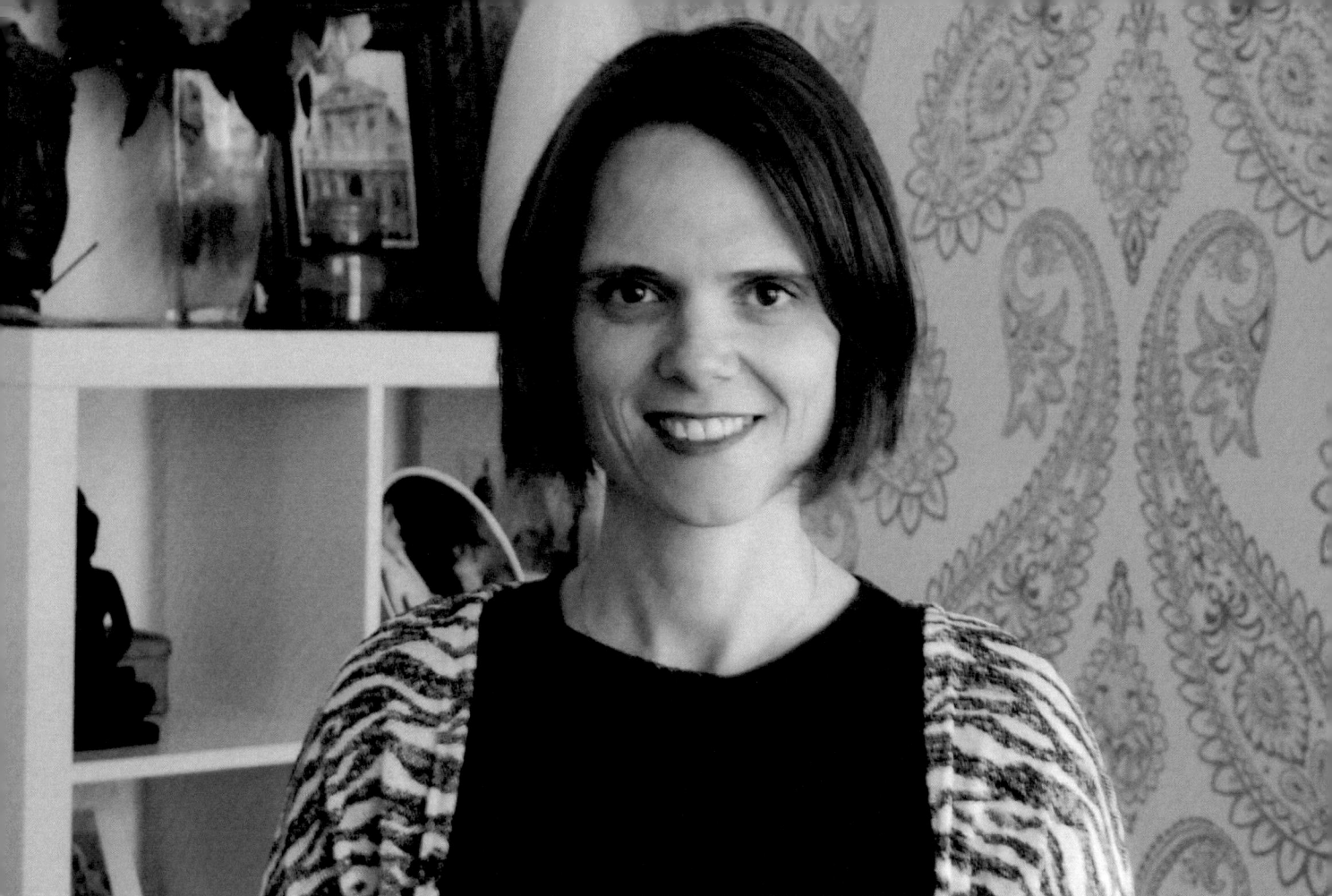

My name is Jennie Williams, I am the director and founder of the user led disability charity, Enhance the UK, and I have degenerative hearing loss. I also have a heart condition called Long QT, which is otherwise known as sudden death syndrome. For communicating, I wear two hearing aids which I rely on a lot. I am also an extremely good lip reader and sign up to British Sign Language (BSL) Level 3. But really, how many people do you know that sign? Within the hearing world, BSL is not much use to me at all.

People tend to get very confused about what hard of hearing actually means. They tend to associate it with old people, so I often get people saying to me, "Oh yeah, my nan wears a hearing aid, we shout at her. I think she has selective hearing...chuckle chuckle." I would be a very rich woman if I had a pound for every time I heard that, and yep, I mean 'heard that' because I can still hear things.

Sometimes, I can be in a room full of wheelchair users at a conference, for example, and I am the most able bodied person there. I am moving tables and chairs, assisting people to the loo if needed, and then speakers will start up on the stage and all of a sudden I am the most disabled person in the room.

I normally can't hear speakers clearly, and often in these circumstances, the hearing loop (if they have one) doesn't work or I can't understand the BSL interpreter (again if they have one) as they are too fast and BSL is not my first language. So I sit, try really hard to lip read, take a painkiller, as I know the dreaded 'hearing headache' will come on, and try my best to keep up. It is hard work trying to lip read and, believe me, I don't know any hard of hearing people who have 'selective hearing.' It depends on someone's tone, how tired you are, your tinnitus (ringing in your ears) and how you feel that day.

When I was growing up I was very embarrassed about my hearing aids, in fact I hated them, and didn't wear them most of the time. I struggled through school trying to be cool and hanging out with the boys at the back of the class but missing out altogether what the teacher was saying. I subsequently failed all my mock exams and scraped through my GCSEs, by having very supportive parents who helped me study at home to try and catch up. Looking back now, I can't honestly say I would have done anything differently. Being part of a group was and is important to me, and I didn't want to isolate myself and be seen as different.

I never really had an issue meeting boys and making friends. My hearing loss was mild at school and so did not come into play much. I was pretty popular and I was able to take advantage of the fact I had a support teacher, Mrs. Simms, sit with me in most classes, taking notes. Poor Mrs. Simms, we all used her notes and rarely did any of our own work!

I was about 21 when my tinnitus became an issue for me. I was living with my first long-term boyfriend and was upstairs getting ready; I thought someone had come in and put the telly on. I knew Simon wasn't home so it really scared me. I went down and of course there was no one there, and the telly was not on. I thought I was going mad and was hearing voices in my head. I talked to my mum and dad about it and my dad explained it was most likely tinnitus, and he suggested I go to the tinnitus clinic. I did, and found it really helpful. I cut out certain foods and stopped drinking caffeine and that helped a bit.

Over the years, my hearing has slowly but surely worsened, and my tinnitus has got louder and louder. When I am at work, I am very assertive most of the time - I have to be. I am a campaigner and a disability awareness trainer – that's what I do. I tell people from the off that I am hard of hearing, and for them to please look at me when they are speaking to me or to keep their hands away from their mouths. I even tell them when I need an eye break. When I am in a social situation however, things can be very difficult and different for me.

I tend to just struggle on a lot of the time: laugh when everyone else is laughing; strain to keep up, and worse still, I apologise. Why is that? I guess I don't want to embarrass people and make them feel like they are not including me. I often feel like I am being annoying when I keep asking what is being said and, frankly, it becomes boring for me as well.

A lot of the time when you say to someone, "sorry"- I always start with a sorry, how very British of me. "Sorry, but I am deaf, could you turn and face me please?" that person will, more often than not, appear to be somewhat embarrassed, say sorry as well and then shuffle around slightly and try to work it all out in their head. You see, I don't seem as though I am hard of hearing. I have a hearing voice as I was born hearing, I am a good lip reader, and you can't see my aids as wear my hair in a bob.
So let's talk about my favourite subject... Dating!

There can be some real perks of dating someone with a hearing impairment; we can get you into the theatre for free or cheap, same with the train, and a lot of us can lip read conversations that you were never meant to know about from quite a way off and get all the gossip. Winning!

Dating someone with hearing loss can be hard and somewhat awkward at times, for all the social reasons I talked about before, not to mention when you are getting down to things and having a good old snog. The last thing you want is your bloody hearing aids whistling every time the hot man (in my mind he is always hot) puts his fingers through your hair, and then your aids end up flying out of your ears onto the floor, and the dog runs in and eats one of them. That is a true story, and it killed the moment I can tell you. I joke about it but I also worry a lot; the person I am now is not the person I am going to end up being. Trying to be intimate with someone when they are whispering sweet nothings in your ear and not be able to hear a thing they are saying is frustrating.

When I was 28 I was in bed with a guy I really liked and had been seeing for a while. He said something to me once I had taken my aids out and the light was off (massive mistake)! I didn't hear him and asked him to repeat himself, he shouted at me saying 'for god sake I am sick of you never hearing me' and rolled over. I didn't sleep that night; I had someone lying in bed with me, that was meant to care about me, and was shouting at me. I finished with him the next morning.

Let me tell you about one of my favourite, and also most awkward, dates. I was single, living in London and looking for a boyfriend, so I did what all single Londoners do – I joined a dating site. I started chatting to this guy who looked cute and we had a bit of banter via email. We soon arranged to meet up as I was not one for chatting online for too long. We met on the South Bank and as I walked out the tube, I was greeted by the cute detective that I had been speaking to. He even looked like like he did in his photos. Result!

We went onto one of the boats on the river and had a drink; we chatted about work, as you do; I may or may not have been twisting my hair and trying to make my lips look all pouty and thinking to myself, 'I really fancy this guy'. So I went to take out my lip gloss and out fell both of my hearing aid batteries. They are really small and so this guy (who I named Gov, as he was a detective and I thought it was funny) said to me, "What on earth do they power?" I then explained my hearing loss and he replied by saying, "why do deaf people do this?" Cut to him waving his hands in the air and scrunching his face up with the tongue in his bottom lip making weird groaning sounds. Oh dear.

I was thinking about throwing my drink in his face but that would have been childish, and a waste of a drink, so I explained about British Sign Language and the culture behind it. I don't think he got it at all but he was embarrassed and didn't know what to say, so he offered to take me for a ride on his massive motor bike (not a euphemism) around London and then buy me dinner.

As a newly single 30 something, with now much worse hearing loss, and tinnitus so bad you want to rip your ears off at times, there is a part of me that really worries about meeting someone who is open minded enough to be ok with it. But it is a part of me and, if I do say so myself, you also get a lot of good stuff as part of the package deal.

So back to the slightly more serious stuff. I started the campaign, Undressing Disability a few years ago. I believe that having a disability can be a very isolating experience. As well as the physical barriers, there is still a huge amount of prejudice towards disability amongst the general public. Whilst working in care homes, I am continually disappointed to see very few people who live there have double beds. This instantly makes you feel childlike and takes away the chance of anyone coming in for a kiss and a cuddle... or god forbid, have sex! Disabled people often say to me they have no-one to talk to about sex and it is still so taboo, especially if you are in the care system and rely on someone to help dress you, feed you and wash you. Your life is not always your own and basic human rights, like being able to have a relationship or simply just have sex, are ignored.

If people want to be sexually active they should be. I think there is this massive misconception that sex workers and disability go hand in hand. In some cases they may, but this should be a choice not the only option that people, men mainly, have. Most people I know and talk to want a loving relationship, and want to feel loved and to love. Everyone has the right to have human touch, even if it is not sex as we know it. Any sense of intimacy between two people who care about one another is so important. Even if it's a one night stand, but it is your choice, that's also important. Let's face it, most of us have not slept only with people we 'love.' We all want to be found attractive, and sexual relationships are the most natural thing in the world.
We set up the Love Lounge, which is a safe place for disabled people and their partners or family members to write in to our non expert sexperts, Emily Yates and Mik Scarlet, for advice about anything from relationships to sexual positions. We had so many people writing in, wanting to tell their stories, we decided to make a book so more people could share their ups and downs, funny and tragic tales alike. We hope you enjoy the read and to know that you are not alone.

End

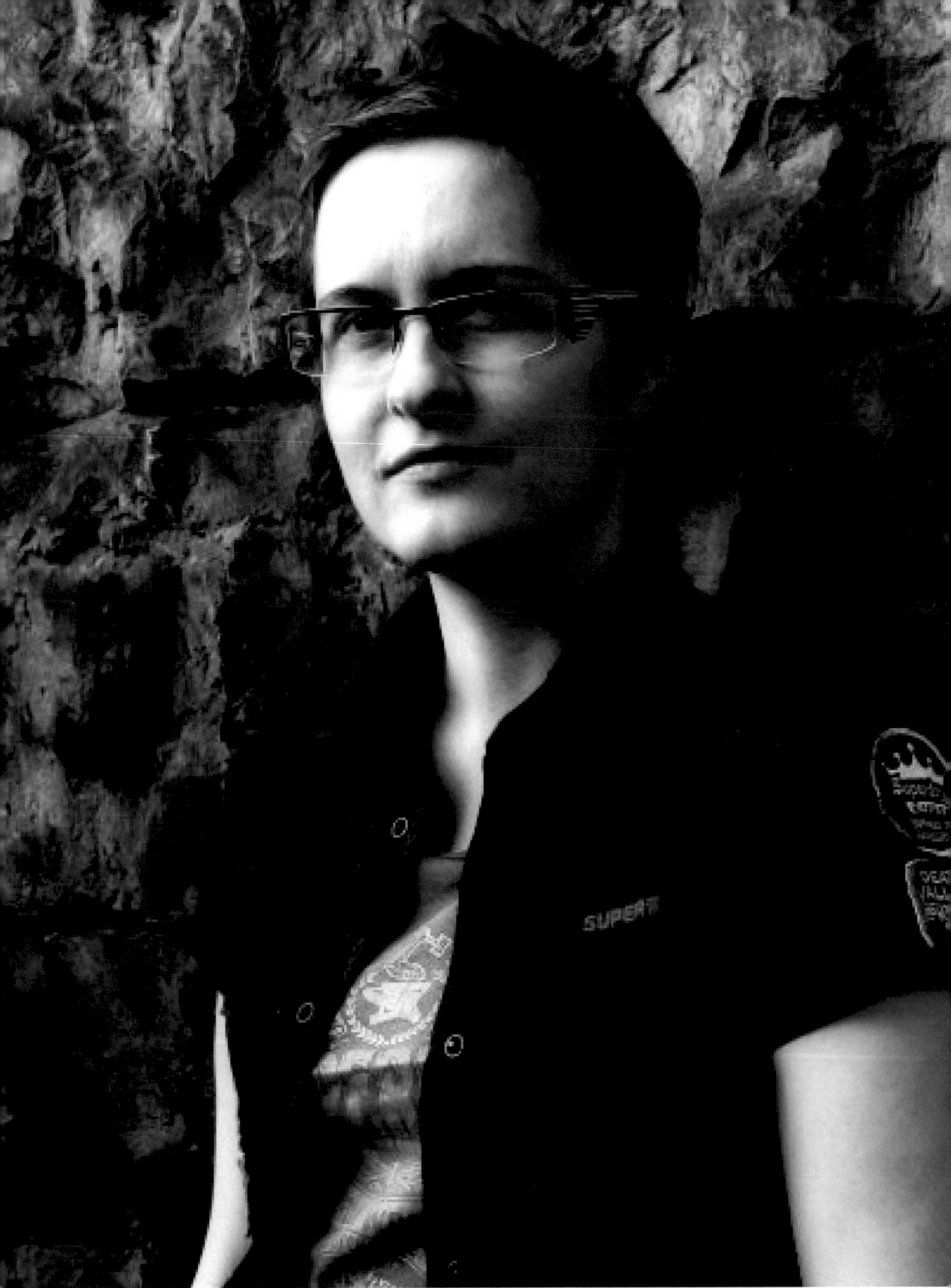

Jacqueline Kelly is a policy and campaigns manager living in Scotland.
Her eyesight is affected by the condition, Retinitis Pigmentosa.

Jacq's story

Scenario 1

There's a party at the house of someone I fake love.

By fake love I mean this:

1. I may love this person
2. I may totally not love this person.

At this stage in our friendship there is, hindsight now shows me, no way I wouldn't really know. This person is someone I barely know when I really think about it. All I really know is that her name is Catherine-Rose, that she is Canadian, and that I fancy the pants off her. I have done since the first time she walked through my kitchen door. She turned up at my flat, which I shared with my then girlfriend, to help us to make pro-choice posters vis-a-vis abortion and was wearing a green jumper and accepted a slice of pizza (not a euphemism) from me - ROMANCE! We then knelt on the carpet and painted wire coat hangers and banners with slogans such as 'a womb of one's own.' This is all true.

I am at the party with this person, who is not interested in me, and a third party suggests I meet her recently single pal for a shag date. I can't see why not, as I'm fairly gung ho. The last matchmaking attempt by a friend of mine was nothing short of disastrous but I'm more than happy to make the same mistake over and over again, so I go for it.

Fast forward a few weeks and I am on my way to meet this friend of the friend of the friend. On arrival, I immediately wonder why I chose one of the darkest basement bars in Edinburgh – I have a condition called Retinitis Pigmentosa, which I'll come to later, but it basically means that I don't see at all in the dark. I find the best lit part of the bar, and finally she arrives. We have a couple of drinks, it all goes well enough, and although it's clear that there is absolutely nothing long-term in this, a couple of weeks later we're back at her place, doing what mildly drunk adults do when there's nothing on the telly.

I am about to acquire my first ever sex related injury and it's all because of the damn eyes. At one point, coming up for air, I misjudge the location of the edge of the bed, which is to say that I simply can't see it so I take a guess. Of course I miss, fly off the actual bed and smack my head on the bedside table. What follows certainly isn't a bloodbath, but this is still, definitely, one of my least smooth moments ever. I am so annoyed at my eyes that I could poke their eyes out, unaware at this point just how much worse things are about to become in the next couple of years.

There are things you don't get told about in life. Sometimes it's because people don't know about them in order to tell you about them, and others it's because there's a degree of taboo attached to it.

When I was around the age of six, our primary teacher took us up the stairs of our old Catholic School to the music room and had us sit around two chairs in a semi-circle. This was exciting stuff, as we knew that we weren't going to be singing today, so something must be afoot. I have a fond memory of the music room – I remember it as a fusty but cosy little cave inside what I otherwise remember as a nice but quite echoey building. I wish I could describe better what happened next, but the truth is that I'd be making it up if I were to elaborate on the basic facts. This was thirty years ago after all, and I wasn't much into journalling at the time. What I do remember is that a man entered the room with a woman who, it turned out, was his wife. He also had a dog. I am going to hazard a guess that, at this stage, we were far more interested in the dog than in its humans. The dog was, you may have guessed, the man's Guide Dog, and he had come to the school to talk to us about his experiences as a blind person and about life with an assistance dog. We were allowed to ask whatever questions we liked (I asked him what he thought the colour red was like) and eventually they pottered away again.

Two things strike me about this now. The first was the absolute way in which we talked about blindness. The man had been blind his entire life and there was no discussion about the fact that many people lose their sight as they progress through their lives and for a range of different reasons. The second is that the role of the man's wife was completely overlooked. To be fair, this is probably because we were a bunch of six and seven year olds and were really more interested in things such as what the man thought the colour red looked like. But I notice that we still don't really talk about either of these things now. In some cases it's because people don't think about it to mention, or they don't know. For others, it's simply an uncomfortable topic that doesn't really bear discussion, unless it really has to be done.

Sitting in that music room, nobody could have told me that from the age of 14, I would start to display the symptoms of Retinitis Pigmentosa because they didn't know – I didn't know, and I wouldn't have a formal diagnosis until the age of 25. But disability was presented to us as a constant – something you would be born with or not. And it feels like, even now, partners are often left out of the discussion, not least when it comes to the impact that another person's disability will have on their lives, or in terms of the impact that disability can have on an intimate relationship.

I was finally diagnosed with RP in 2005 – RP is an inherited condition that leads to a gradual progressive reduction in vision. Difficulties with night vision and peripheral vision are often the first signs of RP, followed by a loss of central vision later on. At the present time, it is the most common cause of sight-loss among working age adults. I'm not the kind of disabled person to be brave about my condition. It pisses me off, makes me angry and stops me doing many of the things I used to love – sport, art galleries, flirting with women to name just a few examples. It's pretty hard to flirt with someone when they have walked away and you've failed to notice because the bar is dimly lit.

Scenario 2

It's the Edinburgh Festival and Edinburgh is jumping with tourists and performers and other groups of people who I also hate. I'm misanthropic at the best of times but the Festival really brings out my inner demon.

There's a woman I have fancied for ages – we'll call her Lena, for that is her name. She's Swedish, and hot, and I like talking to her. Most importantly she laughs at my jokes, and I think that she likes me back. A group at the community centre we both go to usually organise a trip to see the Ladyboys of Bangkok at festival time. This is something I have absolutely no interest in going to, but it somehow comes to my attention that Lena is going along with them, so obviously I get a ticket. I do not look forward to seeing the show, but I do look forward to seeing Lena.

Annoyingly, by the time show time comes around, Lena and I have already got together (high five) but I go anyway. The show turns out to be our second date and although we've known each other for months we are both a bit nervous. For whatever reason, I am in some kind of white cane denial at this stage (possibly due to the cack-handed comments of an ex about not wanting to go out with a blind person) so I leave Old Sticky at home. When we get to the Meadows for the big event I tell Lena something vague about crap night vision, and I ask her if she will come with me to the bar so that I can get us some drinks. She agrees but has no clue what the hell the night blindness thing is all about – fair enough, since I have really failed to explain it at all satisfactorily – she watches on in horror as I walk face first into a wall.

After this I decided that the white stick is going to have to come with us on our dates, and we continue to see each other as a bizarre threesome. Lena gets increasingly better at steering me away from walls/lamp-posts/bins/toddlers/basically everything.

I first became aware that my disability was going to impact on my serious relationships a few years ago – I hadn't even begun to consider this before an on/off shag girlfriend told me that my eyesight was a factor that freaked her out, because she wanted to be with someone who she could enjoy visual things with. You may be able to understand from that why this relationship was usually more 'off' than 'on.' It was something that needled away in my brain over the following weeks, and which came back to haunt me again a few years ago when my current relationship came under some strain, and I faced the prospect of being single again.

The additional obstacles that potentially face a disabled person on the dating scene could merit an entire book of their own, but even within an established relationship, my sight loss creates additional strains that I only become aware of when they impact on me personally. And they go much deeper than accidentally head-butting the bedside table mid-shag. As the world shrinks before my eyes, the number of things I depend on my partner for increases: whether it's finding the thing I dropped on the floor; steering me around people and things or taking on additional household jobs that I find I can no longer do; there's a creeping sense that my partner, Lena, is assuming an increasing number of caring responsibilities.

I first thought about this a couple of years ago at a supermarket checkout. I usually insist on packing the bags (I have OCD tendencies that I have mostly under control, but things like the shopping bags not being packed 'correctly' are likely to torment me until my death) but for some reason I had allowed Lena to do it this one time. I can't tell you now what it was, but there was something in the way that the check-out assistant interacted with us that indicated that they assumed Lena to be my carer. When I asked her about it later, she said that she hadn't particularly noticed anything this time but that she had definitely noticed that, on previous occasions, people seemed to behave as though she was there as a helper of some kind. There are upsides to this: she gets a free ticket on the bus; into the zoo; and into exhibitions at the museum as my 'carer' and we're not going to turn our noses up at saving a bit of dosh. The fact is though, it doesn't feel very sexy. In a similar way, it doesn't scream sexual confidence and dominance when you're having a date night and have to ask someone to hold your hand and take you to the toilet.

It sometimes feels that, as a disabled person, I can't just ask someone to be my partner – I'm always going to be asking them to be something more than just my girlfriend. I'll need them to be patient when I lose my rag after smacking my head for the third time that day; I'll need them to guide me in public spaces; to understand that there are many things I am not going to be able to do with them. When I think about the burden this can put on my partner, I'm often met with denial from friends who mean well, but who insist that of course Lena doesn't mind doing these things for me because she loves me. That's where the taboo comes in. I have no doubt that my girlfriend loves me, but I am also aware that there are aspects of being in a relationship with me that are additionally tiring – actually hardly any of those are a consequence of my disability, but some of them are. Acknowledging that is an important part of any conversation we have about disability and longer term intimate relationships, for the sake of all parties involved.

Scenario 3

I am in a bear bar in Sitges, Catalonia with my girlfriend and some pals. I'm not aware of it at this point, but it's the end of my club-going days. Not because I'm too old – I'm not – but because soon my night vision will be so crap it really won't be worth the stress or hassle of paying a fortune to stand in a dark sweaty noise box. For now though I am just about getting by. The gang are getting drinks at the bar and I am by the dance floor waiting for them to come back. I notice a hottie looking at me, which is nice, but also surprising. I think I'm pretty hot myself, but everyone other than us in here seems to be a big hairy gay fella.

Whatever, I like being flirted at as much as anyone, so I turn to her so say hi. Only then do I realise that I'm chatting my own reflection up – that is in fact a mirror. I feel momentarily sad about my crap eyes, but then instantly better about my undoubtedly impeccable taste.

As my condition progresses I increasingly depend on the people in my life to assume roles that have "caring" elements in them. As a fiercely independent person, I find this difficult to swallow and I'm not getting any better at it. I'm also acutely aware of an additional factor. It's another thing that we aren't supposed to talk about, but I try to live in the real world as much as is possible. We no longer live in times where relationships last until we get old and one of us dies. It is acceptable, even advisable, that when a relationship has reached the point where everyone is more miserable than happy, that it ends.

I hope that doesn't happen and have no real reason to think that it will. But I do wonder how, if it did, I would meet someone else. I loved being single and going out on the pull. I'm good at talking to people and, as a result, was good at chatting them up. In my early twenties I was out most nights and never had problems getting laid dates. I have no idea how I would manage it were I to become single again. RP isn't just taking my sight from me, it's also taking with it my ability to go where I want and do what I want whenever I want. It's also taking a huge chunk of my confidence with it. When Channel 4 aired a dating programme for disabled people called 'The Undateables' there was criticism of the name. I wonder though, how much of that was down to the knowledge that, deep down, many non-disabled people don't consider disabled people to be dating potential, and that the way we do dating really just isn't disabled friendly. That said, while there are obstacles, I have a number of excellent weapons in my armoury. I'm persistent and stubborn as fuck. Additionally, I'm hot as hell. Whatever happens I am, always have been, and will remain, a catch.

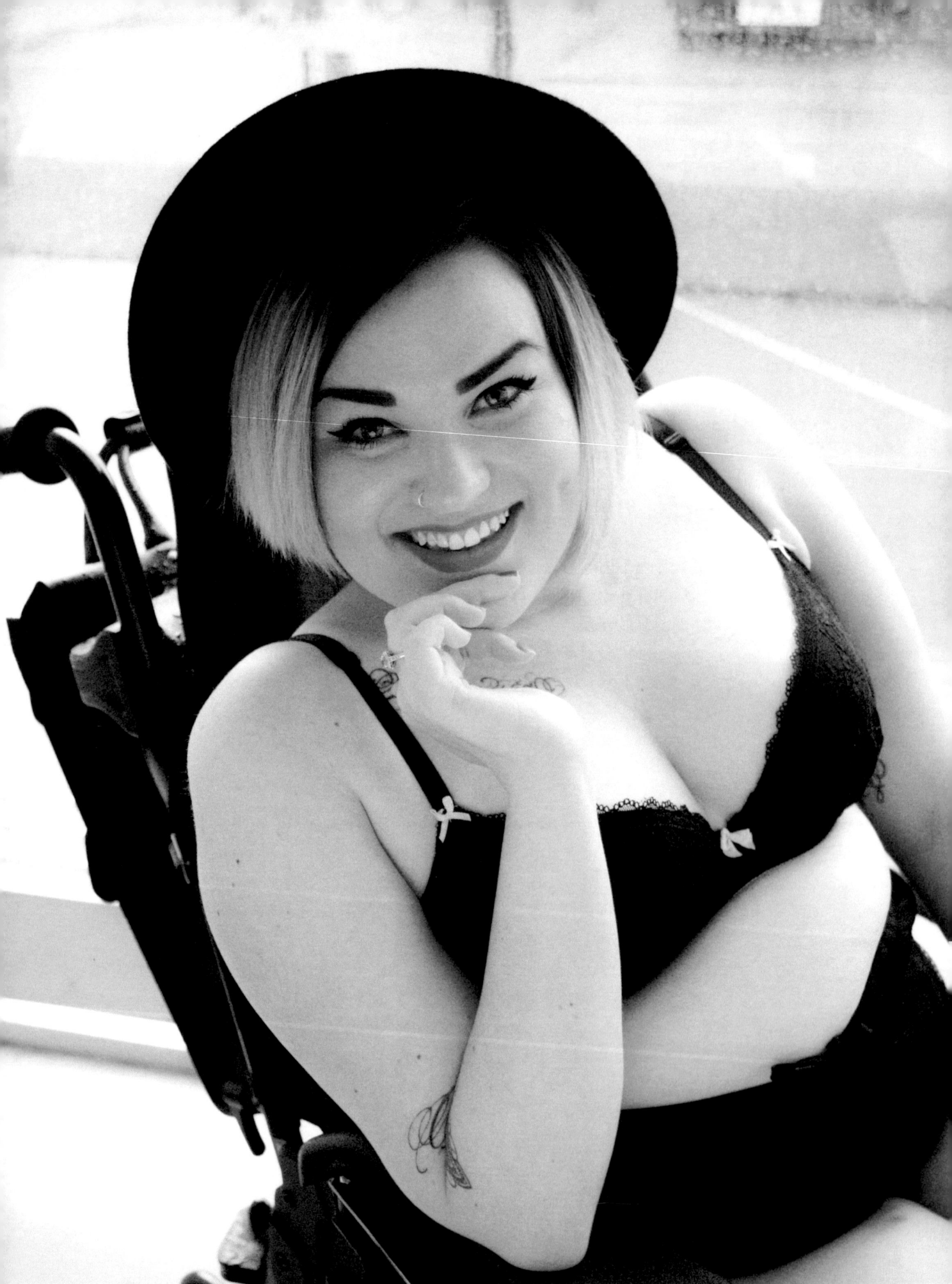

Kelly Perks-Bevington is a 26 year old business owner and blogger.
She has Spinal Muscular Atrophy Type 3 and is a wheelchair user. She is happily married.

Kelly's story

Introduction

I've always shied away from talking about my younger years, for a number of reasons - shyness, irrelevance and just SHEER embarrassment. So when I was presented with this unique opportunity by Enhance The UK, how could I say no?! A chance to talk completely openly about my day to day life, my past and present relationships, and sex.

I'm Kelly, I'm 26 and I have Spinal Muscular Atrophy Type 3 which means that, amongst other things, I use an electric wheelchair on a daily basis. I've never really let the fact that I am disabled affect me, in fact it's probably helped me along the way. It's provided me with the confidence to succeed people's expectations, presented me with some amazing opportunities, and it gives me the chance to constantly surprise people who underestimate me prior to even opening my mouth.

My favourite thing to do is to wait until someone underestimates me, in any situation, and then lay it on really thick, to the point that they are so shocked that they are the ones feeling inadequate and inexperienced. Seriously, once I was at the hairdressers and I was asked by a junior if I'd ever kissed anyone before. I mean, how do you even answer that? I was caught off guard, "why would someone view me like that? Why would that be someone's initial thought when it came to me and relationships? What is wrong with ME?!" I then realised, after a short internal debate, that this person was just SEVERELY uneducated. I then offered them a brief insight into my sexual exploits… and let's just say, that conversation ended shortly after.

I can't complain though, being automatically categorised as innocent DEFINITELY has its upsides, and things have worked out SERIOUSLY well for me in the past because of this. Automatically being discounted from any "bad" situation is obviously an upside, there have been plenty of times where friends of mine have been dragged into police cars, and I am still yet to make that fateful trip to the station (granted, this may have something to do with the lack of police cars with ramped access and space for an electric wheelchair).

The idea of this chapter is to give you all an outline of my past, how I dealt with the awkward teenage fumbles, and how I grew as a person. I must state, I am still "growing", my mind is still expanding, and I still look back at myself last week and wonder, "what the hell was I thinking?!" I am by no means qualified to offer any profound advice regarding dealing with disability in your younger years, but I'll give it a try.

Where it began

When writing, I like to set the scene, so just to give you an idea, now I am perched right on the edge of my wheelchair at the end of my long bench dining table that I brought as a constant source of inspiration. It's meant to fill me with the overwhelming urge to write and create that comes from sitting in a European brunch spot, looking at all of the people, distinctly cooler than yourself tapping away on their iMacs, wearing the most chic, clean, non branded-branded trainers. It doesn't.

I've been procrastinating all day, loading the washing machine, unloading the washing machine, making coffee, eating Snack-a-Jacks. I'm wearing a much loved, very faded, tie-dye shirt; a beanie; no make up; underwear, and some Primarni F-uggs.

When I was younger I was never really sure of what I wanted to be, I was never really confident, and I was certainly never advised regarding sex or relationships. I can't really blame anyone for that. As a kid, I had the best upbringing anyone could ask for. Both of my parents are unbelievably supportive, to the point that they let you make your own decisions and learn from your own mistakes. When I was young, I was never aware of the meaning of my disability and how it really affected me. Of course they explained it to me, but I never saw any boundaries.

I always had a deep routed want to succeed in every sector, whether it was singing in the school play or a running race (literally, on sports day, I did a running race.. and of course I won.. thank god for overly PC primary schools). But seriously, I never took any pride in "winning" anything with assistance, or being praised for something a "normal" person could do with their hands tied behind their back. I didn't want to be pandered to and this made me very defiant, to the point of aggression. I remember numerous occasions where I'd get out of my wheelchair and push it, all the while in my poor little angsty pre-teen brain, thinking a girl hobbling along pushing an empty manual wheelchair looked far more normal than a girl being pushed in a wheelchair. Another moment of this was when I went to a summer camp, I was actually awarded with a certificate on the evening, in front of all of the other kids, for climbing up the stairs to have a shower. I never wanted to be inspirational.

High school

Then shortly after, there was the transition to high school. I was never overtly popular at primary school, but I upheld the "normal" uninteresting kid thing pretty well. Or at least I thought I did.

When I got to high school, I was a train wreck, I had no idea how to act. I had an electric wheelchair that I wasn't used to sitting in; I didn't know anyone; I had massive eyebrows; and I had no idea how to dress my "body"(especially sitting down). I wore an oversized "You'll be able to grow into it" blazer; the worst polyester grey trousers with a crease pressed in all the way down the leg; oh and I still thought the "croydon face lift" ponytail was cool.

The worst thing about moving into secondary school was the sheer size of the school and the fact that they had NO idea how to cater to the needs of a disabled student. I insisted I went to my local school, with no special needs department or assistance. It was great because it paved the way for other kids with disabilities to choose my school, but the things I had to do were actually laughable.

My school was a dual block school, so "A block" was on one side of the road and "C block" was on the other side of the road. They actually made me use a car to get from one side of the road to the other, employing the worst selection of carers to get me to lessons. I had the token, rainbow jumper wearing, patronising carer; the overtly bitchy 'I wouldn't deal with you if I didn't have to' carer; and the just completely momsy carer, that would baby you and snitch out on anything you tried to do. Needless to say, none of them stayed around for very long. But I'm guessing, working with/for a super defiant disrespectful 12 year old wasn't too high on their priority lists either.

I went from this young, angry kid to being an even angrier, bitchier teen. By this time, I'd internally come to the conclusion that I was always going to be patronised, given the benefit of the doubt and basically discounted. I saw myself as some kind of secret cool kid, listening to my battered, bright orange, jumpy portable CD player, half listening to my friends and teachers, all of the time "knowing" that none of them had a clue about what I was capable of.

As most teens do these days, I took to the internet, reinventing myself, talking to guys… and girls - falling in love with everyone and completely baring my soul to all of these people. I still think about them now. I didn't tell anyone I was disabled. I didn't need to.

I was okay looking, with a bit of colour in my hair, a fringe covering most of my face and a token red lip. I spent my time, literally all of my time, talking to these people. I'd take my Dad's whirring, overheating mac to bed with me and I'd stay awake under the covers, chatting to people all over the world, catfish and all. I was completely vulnerable. But I liked it.

The internet literally started my sexual discovery. It was around the time that sex education in schools was completely non-existent and the time where young girls didn't really chat about that kind of thing. I started my education online, chatting about literally anything and everything sex, and it fascinated me. It was addictive.

I then took this knowledge into real life and started mixing with completely the wrong people. I'd found my identity, no-one could patronise me; if they found me sexually attractive and if I had that power over them, or at least that is what I thought. I viewed myself as some kind of superhuman, 'wow I was in a wheelchair and people STILL found me sexually attractive!' It was literally an epiphany and a fantastic excuse for me to treat everyone who loved me like shit.

There was one point where I had most of the local "boys" boarding school on speed dial and I'd regularly speak to one particular dorm room every night, receiving phone calls and explicit text messages. One day my mom unknowingly had a little mess on my phone, supposedly wondering who I was spending most of my time talking to, and was to say the least, shocked. She still talks about that to this day, and safe to say she has never looked at any of our phones ever since.

This completely changed me, I altered conversations within my friend group and stood up for myself, I finally felt like me. I remember, once I came into school with long black and green hair, the teachers were going to make me dye over it, and make me stay in detention. Instead, I "RAN" away. The most hilarious part of this was half way through my attempt to escape, I got a puncture and by the time I got to the bottom of my road my chair was completely on its arse. My nan somehow spotted me, and just as a form of punishment, stopped some builders on the road and got them to push me to the top of our hill. Needless to say, I never attempted to make a break for it again.

I completely took the piss out of my school, using my "physio" room as our lunchtime hang out and smoking spot, and a place I'd hide instead of going to maths. Never getting in trouble, I stopped caring about doing well and I stopped worrying what people thought.

After high school, I basically acted like a Skins cast member - parties, lots of "relationships," lots of underage drinking and smoking and not a care in the world. Occasionally I'd get the, "Get up out of your chair and fight me then" comments. After the first time I actually obliged, realised I was drunk and fell on my arse, I decided to let these comments slide in future.

Speaking of falling on my arse, one particularly cold day, one of the worst things happened to me sex-wise. I was with a "summer fling" at the time, and yes, it was cold in summer, I live in Birmingham! But anyway, we had been out all day doing the usual, and we arrived back at my parents' house, one of my first adapted houses. I always left my wheelchair downstairs, underneath the lift and I'd walk from the lift to my bedroom. I seriously misjudged just how eager I was to get upstairs, and as soon as I got in the lift my freezing legs just gave way! I couldn't get up off the floor with help as I'd never really been with a guy confident enough to suggest a solution, and I guess I was still pretty embarrassed about the whole thing! So I automatically thought of a solution (a stupid one). I sat in the lift and sent myself upstairs, arriving upstairs and then shimming all the way over the landing to the bathroom… I then used the bathroom hoist to lift me to my feet. It was a hell of a lot of effort to go to for something that, let's just say, didn't last very long. View that as you will haha.

College

After the summer came to an end, I was ready to start college. Seeing as my grades weren't great, and I had NO idea what I wanted to do, I ended up on a Media First Diploma course, which is basically the course you go on prior to starting a BTEC. During this time, I met some amazing friends. They were all guys, but they made me feel amazing. None of them saw my disability. They all helped me when we were out, and gave me even more support than any of my female friends did to date. We spent all of our time, between lessons, drinking and terrorising the town that our college was in. God knows how we all didn't get kicked off the course sooner!

It was a very "incestous" group, and we'd spend the rest of our time sleeping with each other or each other's partners. We could be seriously open with each other about EVERYTHING, and this time I felt completely sexually free. Nothing was too weird, it was perfect!

Needless to say, throughout the years, pretty much every avenue was explored. We had group sex, same-sex sex, and none of it felt awkward. My friends, being open and talking about sex daily, helped me express what I wanted and I was never embarrassed. If I needed to be picked up and put on the bed after a few too many JDs, I'd ask!!

However, there were definitely times where I took this new found confidence a little bit too far. Picking up briefly on the previous part, where I spoke about the internet, I actually met a guy online, spent a few days in his company and then decided, in my infinite wisdom, that it'd be a great idea to go out in my car to a country lane lay-by, have a few drinks and "sleep" in the back of my converted car. It wasn't until after I got onto the floor of the car that I realised, I actually didn't know this guy very well, I had no way of standing up on my own without his help and I could've possibly put myself in the most dangerous position I'd ever been in. Luckily he turned out to be a really nice guy and everything was absolutely fine, we actually ended up together for a long time after that. But the point is, that it could have gone a completely different way!

During college, after a lot of messing around, I got into a long term relationship but it was still just as fun. We still included other people in our relationship as optional extras. We spent a lot of time with my friends, going out, and things finally seemed to have taken a relatively normal turn. The trouble is, with normality, I seem to get bored quite easily and, as I mentioned before, I also have a tendency to fuck things up.

Ultimately, things ended.

Getting serious and growing up

Following various relationships and focusing seriously on my career, things began to level out. I was in a good job, I had a car and a social life. However, I was missing a little bit of my past, I missed my carefree college days, I missed my friends, the ones who moulded me, the ones who gave me the confidence to do all of these things!

A part of the story I missed out is that our closest friend, the friend who glued all of the pieces together, actually passed away really suddenly, when we were nineteen. It shook our friend group to the core and we actually went our separate ways instead of coming together. I don't know why, all I know is, it was definitely the wrong thing to do.

I won't talk anymore about our friend, because.. I don't think I can or should, but it was time to reach out to Jaz, one of the five of us who I had a very special relationship with. Although, in our younger years, we could never commit and we were always at each other's throats, and competing with each other, we'd stay awake on the phone all night, have private coffee dates and secret sleepovers. I missed him so much. So one day I reached out, and before I knew it we were on another coffee date together and things had gone completely back to normal.

With Jaz, our relationship has never been smooth-sailing. We are both stubborn, competitive and sometimes bloody stupid, and it took a while to get it right, but he still keeps me on my toes. I still get butterflies when he texts me - even though we are now married, and have a house together. He makes me better myself, he gives me the confidence I had when I was that college girl, and he drives me to succeed. The point is, with Jaz I don't miss anything. I sit with him, knowing that he was the person that was missing in my life for so long. He IS my ambition and drive. I get as much enjoyment going out clubbing, the two of us, as I would from going out with an entire group. We bounce off each other, and we have the best sex because we love each other. We know each other completely, and we can be totally honest with each other.

I think if I had one piece of advice for someone/anyone who wants it, it would be, in sex.. and life, if you need help, ask for it, if you want to try something go for it. Take risks, no matter who you are, and always challenge yourself. Always try to be better, always try to be happier and always search for the person/people that make you want to live and achieve.

David Ward is 23, originally from Runcorn and now living in London.
He currently works as a Recruitment and Selection Officer for The Future Leaders Trust,
selecting the most able teachers that can make a difference in challenging schools.
He is passionate about LGBT and disability rights.

David's story

I guess a good place to start would be to explain what I'm doing in this book. I have amniotic band syndrome (ABS), which has caused – without wanting to get too medical about it – disfigurement and stunted growth of my limbs and digits. Essentially, in the womb, bands wrapped around my extremities and constricted their proper growth. What this means at a basic level is that one of my legs is shorter than the other one (not hugely noticeable) and some of my fingers are more stumps than fingers (slightly more noticeable). Although a relatively rare condition, I have managed to stumble across a checkout girl at the Asda in my town who also has ABS. A girl I sat next to in a class at college - now one of my best friends - also happened to have a 'tiny hand', as she called it. Whilst it does affect my day-to-day life significantly, with the expected slowness with typing and writing, pain when walking and other mobility problems, where it has had a more insidious effect is on my self-esteem. Being marked out as an 'other' by my classroom assistants, extra time in exams, and constant doctor and physiotherapy visits likely instilled in me an acute awareness of my own disability and how it permeates my daily life.

As stupid as this might sound, I grew up expecting rejection from people due to my hands – especially in future relationship terms. My mum has always maintained that people do not care and that I shouldn't be so worried, but fears like that aren't something a mother can easily brush aside. First-hand experience is what counts when it comes to your self-esteem in regards to these things. Besides, mum can bring out the 'I told you so' far into the future, on my wedding day or engagement or whatever other time she sees fit. My fears of rejection were made more frightening by the fact that I was gay. Gay and disabled was something that I just didn't see as compatible, I had never even heard of a gay and disabled person before. Gay men were judgemental! Gay men were obsessed with appearance! None of them would want to be with someone with such obvious disfigurements! And thus my hyperbolic doom-laden thought process continued down this path for a while.

When I actually got a boyfriend, during my first year of university, I spent the first week or so worrying about it. Did he know? Was he too polite to ask? Did he think they were weird and was trying to ignore it? When I eventually plucked up the courage to approach the subject, incidentally in the most inopportune moment I could have picked - lying on top of him on his bed in the middle of making out - it turns out he had already noticed and didn't care at all. We were together for another two and a bit years after that. Point one to mum.

My second relationship actually began with me straight out telling the guy about my fingers – in the middle of the date and after a significant amount of making out, naturally. I think I was trying to force the issue to stop the same anxiety I had felt in the beginning days of my first relationship. And from then on, when meeting people on Grindr, after moving to London, if I go on a date with someone I usually play it by ear and see if they mention it. Only a few of my many dates (I'm 22 and in London, don't judge me) have actually brought it up – and all of these have maintained that it isn't a problem and that it is quite cute. Although this is meant as flattering and I do take it as such, in the back of my mind I feel somewhat infantilised by this. Are my hands cute because they are small and child-like? Does it mean I need looking after? Still, when it comes to my previous worries about never finding anyone, I'd much rather be a little patronised than forced into the celibacy I had imagined as a drama queen adolescent. No-one has, as of yet and to my face, turned me down or been disgusted by my hands. They definitely haven't hindered me when it comes to after the date either. I might struggle to take lids off jars but my grip is perfectly fine in the bedroom.

One date has definitely stayed in my memory though: it was perfectly pleasant, we had things in common, and enjoyed a few fancy beers. Afterwards, during the pre-requisite post-date instant messaging, he said something which really hit me: 'You don't have to hide your hands, you know'. I realised he was referring to the way I hold my drinks, an exaggerated and somewhat awkward pose that hides my fingers as much as possible. Not only is this probably drawing more attention to them and so is very counter-intuitive, but it's also taking up a lot more of my thoughts than it needs to. I need to be able to be honest with the men I see, and with myself, about my disability. Some of the men I've seen still might not know about my hands – though during sex, when they go to grab my hands, surely they must tell some fingers are amiss? Maybe they just think I'm really angry or on edge. Either way, I need to learn to let go and enjoy myself in the moment, without worrying about what others might think of my hands. It's a tough thing to achieve, but I'm trying.

It appears that, big surprise, gay men are just like everyone else. I'm sure there are some men who I could meet on a date who would think less of me because of my hands, but equally, there are people who contested my family using a disabled parking space as a child, or people who stare at my hands on the tube, with some kind of morbid fascination. People can be awful, but they can also be wonderful and accommodating. My message to other LGBT people who have a disability is to remember that you are not alone in this, and you are not invisible. We are out there, and we do have sex, go on dates and have relationships. The world of dating isn't perfect for us and some people might treat us differently, but don't let it put you off – go out and enjoy life. Everyone deserves that.

E's story

First of all, let me start by saying that I am now in a happy fulfilling relationship with a guy who is not deaf but accepts me for who I am. Like everyone, I am sure, the road to true love has been rocky. In fact, that's a bit of an understatement.

I suppose my story really starts when I was seven years old and was diagnosed as deaf. I had no hearing in my right ear and was moderately deaf in my left ear.

Back in those days (nearly 30 years ago I hate to admit) there was no such thing as the newborn hearing screening and therefore it was not uncommon for kids to slip through the net. My mum frequently brought to my school's attention that she was sure something was wrong with my hearing, and therefore I was called in to do another hearing test. It was like a game to me. The problem was that I have always hated to fail. Every time I heard a sound I was praised and that was just the kind of attention I wanted. So when I couldn't hear a sound, it was easy to conclude that when the lady (with big bushy eyebrows) pressed the button, so should I. Needless to say I passed every hearing test. Eventually, a substitute teacher decided herself that there was something not right with my hearing, and I was referred to my local hospital. My mum must have looked like a complete moron punching the air, exclaiming "Yes, Yes, Yes," during that conversation with the teacher. I was most upset to realise that I could not cheat (although I saw it as being resourceful) my way through this particular hearing test. My time at the hospital was a bit of a blur and I simply remember sitting in the car on the way home, crying because I was no longer normal.

I was fitted with a hearing aid in my left ear a few weeks later - it was pointless wearing one in my right ear. I hated it with a passion. There was none of this being eased in gently. My parents decided that if I wore it all the time I would get used to it quicker. It was painful to start with, and the headaches were horrendous. I was literally overwhelmed with sounds that I didn't know existed. I vividly remember going into a public toilet and hearing the lady next door having a wee. I was mortified and, strangely enough, always did my best to avoid public toilets for years afterwards. Worse than the headaches and the blisters on my ears though, was the embarrassment of having my hearing aid on show. At the time, it felt like I was wearing a neon flashing sign saying 'not normal.' This wasn't helped by the attempts of my family to make me feel better. "You're still beautiful even with a hearing aid," or the jokes, "You should lend it to Granddad; he could make use of it." I was extremely jealous of my twin sister at this point and actually quite bitter. She was the one who was supposed to have problems with her ears, not me (she had to have grommets fitted earlier on and was now able to hear perfectly).

Ingrained in my memory is when my teacher, I assume attempting to be helpful, informed the class of my hearing loss. I was made to stand at the front of the class, where it was explained that I couldn't hear properly and that I had to wear a special aid to help me. The class was instructed to be nice to me, as it wasn't my fault that I couldn't hear and wasn't the same as everyone else. I wanted the ground to swallow me whole. It doesn't take a genius to conclude that I was badly bullied straight after this. Kids can be cruel and they certainly were. During games of kiss chase it was always, "ahh the deafo is gonna catch me ... Noo." I quickly stopped taking part in playground games and became introverted.

It was drummed into me by my parents that it was a cruel world, and that I had to be strong enough to compete with others who did not have my disability. My dad's mantra was that to succeed in life I would have to be the best at everything, otherwise I wouldn't stand a chance. If I dared to come home with a B grade his first question was, why had I not received an A, and how could I make sure I did next time. I certainly believed everything he said, and dedicated my time to being the best I could at everything. In short, I became a swot. However, the problem with seeking perfection is that you can never be good enough. Whilst doing me a favour academically, it certainly didn't help my social skills. I was so incredibly shy, I didn't have any friends except for my sister's, who tolerated me. She was always the 'social one' and I was the 'clever one'. Things were tough at home as well, with my mum suffering from severe depression and often becoming violent. To cope with everything, I simply withdrew into a fantasy world where a magic wand would be shaken and I would be hearing and normal again, and when I wasn't daydreaming I was reading everything I could get my hands on.

My mum certainly never accepted my deafness. It wasn't unusual during one of her many low days to hear her blame herself for it. It was my dad who got stuck in and was proactive about supporting me. He became heavily involved with the local Deaf Children's Society and eventually became chairperson. Regular events were organised, which I attended with my sister, for example Christmas parties. I remember being so excited about meeting other people like me, who would understand me. I was finding it more and more uncomfortable being with large groups of hearing people as I simply couldn't follow what was being said. My hearing continued to deteriorate and I was now profoundly deaf. It had reached the point where I would miss half of the majority of conversations. Not wanting to look stupid, I would do what I call the nodding dog routine: nod my head and smile at times that I thought might be appropriate, and hope to God that I didn't look stupid.

Unfortunately, the hope that I would fit in with others who understood me was soon crushed. The events were always very awkward for me. The majority of the other kids used British Sign Language and I didn't. This meant I couldn't communicate with most of the kids there, and spent my time talking to the adults. I vividly remember feeling that I simply didn't fit in. Things did improve when we moved house and I attended a school that had a Hearing Impaired Department. Slowly, I started to pick up signing and be able to communicate in BSL. I still never felt at home with deaf people though, and considered myself to be an outsider.

As I navigated the awful teenage years, my self-confidence decreased further. I was a very frumpy teen with terrible short hair, braces and huge plastic glasses, in contrast to my sister who had lovely long hair, didn't wear glasses and who was a hit with the boys due to her curvy figure and flirty manner. As for flirting, I didn't have a clue. I became known as the ice queen, mainly because, regardless of what hurtful things were said, I never showed any emotion or response. This was my way of dealing with things and it served me well, both at home with my mum and at school. I wasn't bullied any more, as it just wasn't fun for them, and I was no pushover. Throughout the school, people identified me as the deaf twin. I hated it, as my deafness was not part of my identity then.

My mum picked up on the fact that I wasn't comfortable in either world – the deaf or hearing - and I have never forgotten a conversation we had whilst washing up, when I was about 14. "I worry about whether you will ever find a boyfriend," she said. I looked at her in puzzlement. "Let's face it, no hearing guy is going to want you as you are damaged goods and no deaf guy will want you as you are not really deaf," she continued. I stared at her and simply walked up to my bedroom to reflect upon what she said. The more I thought about it, the more I thought she was probably right.

You might ask what all of this has got to do with relationships and sex. I think it is important that you understand the impact that my hearing loss had on me. I believe that the low self esteem that I had, and the lack of personal identity, and feeling that I was 'damaged,' not normal and unworthy, in turn fed into the relationships that I ended up in.

I was a really late starter when it came to boys. I didn't have my first kiss until I was 17. He was a mate of my sister's boyfriend, and we were out in a club with a group (it was so much easier to drink underage then). I was a little in awe of him as he was well over six foot tall and blonde, and therefore ticked my criteria of being fit. He was also 22, so I assumed he was well out of my league. At some point during the night, whilst attempting to dance on the sticky floor, in a smoky dark corner of the room, he started whispering in my ear. Oops, never a good move trying to do that when communicating with a deaf girl. I pushed him away and focused on his lips. He asked, "What would you do if I kissed you?" I would like to say that I said something really flirty like "why don't you try it and find out?" but unfortunately that wasn't the case. After turning bright red, I managed to stutter, "I don't know," and ran to the toilets. I spent the rest of the night kicking myself about it. As it turns out, all was good in the end. He was staying at ours and we ended up having a drunken snog on the living room floor. I was so embarrassed, after assuming that he couldn't possibly have actually wanted to kiss me, and his behaviour was obviously fuelled by alcohol, that I hardly ever said two words to him after that.

There was a bit of a pattern when it came to mates/ brothers of my sister's boyfriends for a while. Next there was the best mate of the new boyfriend. He was a complete idiot and I worked with him. He had found out I was a virgin, and spent weeks chatting me up every time he saw me. Luckily, I was too shy to take him up on it, as it turns out that he had been dared to 'pop my cherry.' I was really humiliated when I found out. He actually had the gall to turn round and say, "you didn't really think I could find someone like you attractive did you?" That was really the one to help my confidence. Then there was the brother of the next boyfriend. He actually did like me; he started turning up at college to walk me home and became stalkerish. My sister and I were living by ourselves at this point, as things had got so bad at home. One night we had been to a party and he stayed at ours. I woke up in the middle of the night to him trying to get into my bed. After telling him to get lost, I eventually took pity on the fact that he was sleeping on the floor and told him he could sleep in my bed if he kept his hands to himself. He woke me up in the middle of the night saying he couldn't sleep as he had an itch he couldn't scratch. No, this wasn't a code for something else; he actually did ask me to scratch his back. The problem was that when I gave his back a good scratch, his breathing started to become heavier. In my naivety I didn't realise what was happening and carried on. Literally, within seconds, he rolled over; grabbed my nightshirt; ripped it off; and came in his pants! To say I screamed is an understatement. My sister, and his brother, came running in and escorted him out of my room. I avoided scratching anyone's back for a long while after that!

Things continued in this way right the way through college. I had been studying hard and working pretty much full time to support us. It was an expectation that I would achieve good grades, and towards the end I crumbled under the pressure and went off the rails a bit. I stopped studying and started going out all night, drinking. This might not sound like a big deal to you, but remember that I was a goody two shoes who wouldn't even consider talking to someone in class or not doing my homework. It was at this time I got together with my first boyfriend. He was gorgeous, and obviously experienced. I felt so incredibly lucky that he would even look at me twice, that I put up with the fact that conversation with him was as stimulating as watching paint dry. We never actually had sex (I always thought there must be something wrong with me) and, after spending a fortune on presents, he dumped me on Valentine's Day. Luckily the time spent in the back of his car at the airport didn't hamper my attempt to get good grades!

Everything changed when my sister and I left the flat and went our separate ways to Uni. I was still living in my hometown, as the London Uni I attended had taken so long to assess my needs regarding support that it was too late to secure a room in the halls, and I couldn't afford anything else. I should have realised then, that my first foray into Uni was doomed. I suddenly understood that I wasn't able to cope in a lecture theatre environment without communication support. Although I was entitled to it, it simply didn't happen. The Uni was shockingly poor with the support that they offered. Up until this point, other than socially, I had always been able to achieve anything that I decided I should. It hit me, that my disability could and would limit things that I could do. I didn't have the confidence to stand up and fight the university, and accepted their stance that they simply couldn't find support. I left within a year. Interestingly, it was about this time that I started to gain confidence in myself as a person. I could no longer hide behind my sister and rely on her for a social life. I got to the point that I realised that I was so guarded that no-one actually knew me for who I was. I decided that if one person could like me for me then I would be happy. I started to come out of my shell a bit, and I noticed that people started to look at me in a different way. I actually had friends of my own, and this made me feel so much happier. There were still times, of course, when I struggled to cope with groups or missed what was being said but I handled it better.

I finally lost my virginity, with my second boyfriend, at the age of nearly 19. I would like to say it was a fabulous experience but I would be lying. Again, he was older and I actually felt grateful that he was interested in me. The fact that he was a perpetual liar was simple to overlook, as was his temper, until he punched me in the face for saying he was being pathetic. He did this in the street, and when a group of youths saw him and had a go at him, which resulted in him getting a slap, it was me who was to blame. I was shaken, upset and tearful, and that was the end of that relationship.

I don't intend to bore you with details about every relationship that I have ever entered into but the next one was probably the most important of my life in some ways, as I have my gorgeous son out of it. It was also the worst relationship I have ever been in. I met Paul at work. Again, he was tall and blonde and I thought he was gorgeous. All the women at work fancied him, as did I. My stomach would literally flip every time I saw him. He had a natural charm about him and was very easy going. I think this was one of the main things that attracted me to him. We became good friends, and I expected it to stay at that. Eventually, he asked me out on a date. I turned up incredibly nervous at the local pub where we had agreed to meet. He forgot his wallet and so I ended up paying for everything (that should have been a warning).

I fell pregnant the first time I slept with him. We had used condoms and I had taken the morning after pill but it was obviously meant to be. To say this put pressure on our relationship was an understatement. He agreed to stand by me, and things became serious very quickly. He was going through a very difficult time himself. He had Crohn's disease and had to have major surgery to remove part of his colon and have an ileostomy. This meant that he had a bag fitted to his small intestine, which was sticking out of his abdomen to collect his poo. This would give his large intestine a chance to rest and recover. He was often in a great deal of pain and in and out of hospital. He was also battling personal demons of his own regarding his family, and was really depressed. My pregnancy wasn't easy. I was 19; in and out of hospital; my partner was really poorly; and we literally had nothing. Our beautiful son was born, and within a week Paul was threatening to leave me. He said he couldn't cope with how things had changed, and said that he felt pressured into being a dad. He also suggested that I give our son up so we could spend time just the two of us. Obviously this wasn't going to happen. Due to financial reasons I had to return back to work full time when my son was just six weeks old, as Paul was only able to work part time due to his ill health. We had our ups and downs but decided to get engaged. We bought our own flat and settled into life.

Things slowly started to change between us. I couldn't put my finger on what it was, but it started by Paul getting angry quickly and shouting in my face. It quickly progressed into him calling me all kinds of names and telling me how lucky I was to have someone like him, as I was impaired. Unfortunately it wasn't just my hearing that was impaired at this time, but also my thinking. I would always make excuses for him, and blamed myself for not being good enough for him. It then slowly progressed into a push or a shove and things being thrown in my direction. Every time something like this happened it was like a bit more of my spirit got thrown with it. Looking back it was clearly an abusive relationship right then, and yet if anyone had said this to me I would have just denied it. It ended up becoming very violent. The sex was terrible, I didn't feel attractive and the focus was always on pleasing him and keeping him happy. At this point, I still didn't know what an orgasm was. The more I tried to make him happy and be like a porn star the less he cared about how I felt or how it was for me. One night I must have annoyed Paul more than normal and he decided he would teach me a lesson. He dragged me by the hair into the bedroom, pushed me down and raped me anally. I struggled but that just hurt even more so eventually I just lay there, silently crying. I couldn't believe what had just happened. It took me a long time to even acknowledge that it was rape. This still wasn't enough to make me leave him. We separated briefly a few times when he left me, but I always had him back.

My family was oblivious to all of this, until one night I couldn't keep it from them. Paul and I were out celebrating my 21st birthday (late as he had left me on my birthday). He became very drunk and decided to accept some cocaine that was offered to him. It didn't take long for things to turn sour. By the time we were home he slapped me about quite a bit. He had eventually left and I had locked the door on him and refused to open it. Eventually he knocked on the window and I lip-read him telling me that he was in agony and needed to use the toilet. Considering his Crohn's disease, I opened the door and let him in. This was a big mistake. He pushed me into the corner and tried to throttle me. He then punched me and threw me across the room resulting in me being knocked out and left unconscious whilst he trashed the flat and walked out, leaving me there. When I came to, I was so disorientated and couldn't breathe. I ended up phoning my dad, who took me to hospital. Luckily, my son was at his other grandparent's house. I refused to tell the hospital who was responsible, much to my dad's disgust, and ended up being stitched. It was painful for days but the worst part was the emotional turmoil. He had literally smashed most of the things we had owned, and every time I looked around I was reminded of the state my life was in. I didn't allow him back for a long time after that; only agreeing, when he sought help for his temper. I would like to say that this was the last time but it wasn't. Our relationship eventually ended when he decided to pin me down and hold a knife to my throat. Our son had woken up and toddled through. He saw what was happening and started to cry, and come towards me. Paul picked him up and threw him. Eventually I managed to persuade him to let me get up and sort out our son.

You might ask why I have told you all of this. It angers me when people say how only weak stupid people put up with abusive relationships. Looking back I was incredibly vulnerable, with such a low self-esteem that I was an easy target. I generally believed that it was my entire fault, and if I could just be better things would be ok. I became deeply depressed and felt that I would always be alone as a single mum, and that I would never find anyone who would really love me. My son was my saving grace during this period. I loved him with all my heart and had to keep on getting up in the morning and going to work for him. Eventually I picked myself up and hit the dating scene again.

As I grew older, I started to accept my deafness more. I realised that it was and is an essential part of who I am. I started to date deaf guys, something which I had not previously done before. I spent more time around other deaf people, and finally started to feel like I belonged in the Deaf community. I attended (and still do) deaf events all around the country. I realised, finally, that I didn't have to belong solely in one world but could belong in both (the deaf and hearing), and that I was in a lucky position. I suppose, in short, I developed my own sense of identity. I was no longer embarrassed, and instead became proud of who I am. I no longer wished that I could be hearing, and felt a sense of peace about myself.

Dating deaf guys had its advantages and disadvantages. They didn't assume I fancied them purely because I happened to look at their faces. I never had to worry about not understanding what was being said or having to concentrate on lip-reading when I was tired. I didn't have to explain my deafness, and it was seen as an advantage that I was deaf and not a disadvantage.

Deaf sex, especially when both people involved are deaf can be funny. There is certainly no turning the lights off if you want to communicate. I soon learnt, whilst he is 'down there' pleasuring you with a bit of oral, to keep quiet and your hands still - otherwise it all stops right at the wrong moment while he pops up and asks you what you said! There's nothing quite like dating a deaf guy who lives with his parents and having to have sex against the door to ensure that no one knocks and enters without you hearing. How I nagged about getting a lock fitted, but it soon became like a game. You would be amazed about how many positions you can do against a door. You're more susceptible to getting caught in the act too. It dampens the passion somewhat when you have a security guard shining his light on you, and all you can see is the light shining on your partner's backside when you decide to have a quickie in the woods. It seems that his shouting at us had failed to grab our attention so he went and got the flashlight. Then there's the time we were having a session in the shower. Caught up in the moment, he had forgotten to remove his hearing aid and, when realising that it was getting drenched, jumped out of the shower, slipped over and badly sprained his wrist.

Deaf sex is also never quiet, as my hearing friend found out to her detriment. On attending a camping event for deaf people, we were chilling in the tent when a look of horror appeared on her face. When asking what was wrong, she explained that she could hear a couple having sex, then another one and then another. At one point she didn't know where to look. I woke up bright and breezy the next morning. She on the other hand looked like death warmed up. She explained that listening to the bloke who sounded like a lion roaring, and the other who sounded a bit like a steam train all night, was not her idea of fun. Funnily enough she hasn't attended another deaf camping event since then.

There are disadvantages of dating within the Deaf community. I have only ever properly dated or been in relationships with four deaf men. One of whom lived in London, another who lived in Sheffield, one who lived in Scotland and the final one lived near Cambridge. I met these guys at different times through different channels and didn't know that they had anything in common. Yet one evening found myself in the unfortunate position of being sat down at a table at a deaf event in Bournemouth to find all of them sat at the same table. Now that simply wouldn't happen with hearing guys.

It would be wrong to portray all the hearing guys I have dated as bad men who were detrimental to my mental wellbeing. I have been out with some lovely guys, one of whom I was with for several years and continue to be very close friends with. It simply didn't work out, mainly due to the age difference. He was 20 years older than me and we eventually wanted different things in life. There is a deep-seated friendship and respect there, which I hope will never be broken.

It would also be wrong to assume that the reason the guys who didn't treat me well were like this because of my deafness. I genuinely don't think it had anything directly to do with my hearing loss. I set the bar in the relationships that I entered by not having a good sense of self worth and accepting the treatment that was dished out. I was so desperate to be loved and felt unworthy of it that I accepted 'love' in whatever form it was given. As I have grown as a person and accepted myself for who I am, I have raised that bar.

I am now in a loving relationship with the most thoughtful romantic man. Don't get me wrong, he isn't perfect but then who is? He treats me and my son with love and respect; makes us both laugh; and we have a healthy sex life, which is important. I can't say that my deafness doesn't impact on our relationship at all. He is a Northerner, so at times when he speaks to me, I struggle to understand him and have to ask him to slow down. He has agreed to learn BSL, as communicating with me in the mornings can be difficult and I can become especially grumpy. It will also allow him to be fully included in my life which involves meeting lots of deaf people, and attending deaf events. He is keen to do this, and has thrown himself head first into it. He does at times struggle to understand the different culture. For example, he finds how tactile deaf people are just strange.

I am always aware that at times he does support me in ways he wouldn't have to with a hearing girl. For example, if we are out and about he will alert me to sounds I don't hear and he will often make telephone calls for me or if I can't understand someone he tells me what they are saying. At times I have worried about this. He didn't sign up to our relationship to become a 'carer.' Then I sit down and put things in perspective. I realise that I help and support him in lots of ways too and that I shouldn't get hung up about these things. When looking at my relationships and sexual experiences since that very first kiss, I realise that they tell a lot about where I was in my acceptance of my deafness. It is only since I have fully accepted myself for who I am that I have had positive experiences. It's an old saying but I think it's appropriate – you can't expect anyone else to love you if you can't love yourself.

Conor and Shelbi's story

How we met

I'm Connor and I recently turned twenty, which was pretty weird. Before moving to University in Salford I'd lived in the same small town my whole life. None of the buses are wheelchair accessible, so I'd have to rely on lifts from my Mum, which could be pretty embarrassing but my mum is pretty cool. The main streets are cobbled which is hell for any wheelchair-user, but the people are friendly and most of my friends and family are there.

My secondary school could be a nightmare at times, they wouldn't bother to fix lifts or arrange accessible transport for school trips a lot, which made me feel invisible at times. If it wasn't for my friends and a handful of helpful teachers I probably would've hated school. The thing I love to do more than anything else is playing the drums and whenever I tell people this, a lot of them have the same reaction of disbelief; 'How on Earth could someone in a wheelchair possibly play drums?!' is maybe what they think. I play in a band and we take what gigs we get, which can sometimes mean drunken band mates carrying me up and down flights of stairs, but that's something to go in my autobiography when I'm a rockstar. I love films of all kinds, and my dream job would be to write for the screen. I like a lot of geeky stuff too; I have a lot of comics and Videogames, and I can name some pretty obscure Star Wars characters (something I'm oddly proud of). Now we get to my disability. I've never been fully diagnosed, something which doesn't really bother me too much, although it does make filling in any medical forms even more of a hassle. My condition is a congenital, neuromuscular disorder (various muscular dystrophies and myopathies have been ruled out over the years) and has stayed pretty much the same my whole life, and probably won't change in the future. I use a manual wheelchair full-time, and this can be frustrating at times; arranging to go most places takes extra effort with checking accessibility, and sometimes strangers will choose to use it as a conversation starter when they could pick literally anything else. When I was around ten I had Titanium rods screwed onto my spine to stop it from curving further, as I had scoliosis. I remember my Dad was caught by the police speeding to see me on his motorbike after the operation. I was meant to spend two weeks in hospital and I spent just over one (I've always been a jammy git). Sure I'll never get to climb Mount Everest or trip over my own shoelace, but I think having a disability has given me a perspective on life that not many people have. Being disabled feels like being in an elite club, just one that has to have its clubhouse on the ground floor.

I met Shelbi at a disability sports camp at Stoke Mandeville when I was thirteen, and although it was a sports camp I was mainly there to socialise. I played various sports but I was never really the competitive type as I was too nice to have that 'killer instinct'. The fact that I have never been diagnosed also meant that it was near impossible to classify me if I had chosen to play sports competitively. A close friend of mine introduced me to Shelbi and I immediately liked her, and remember spending as much time with her as I could (without it being considered stalking), and although we always hung around in a big group of our friends I was always drawn to Shelbi.

We met every year at these camps for a while, but to begin with we lost touch in the intervening months. Eventually, I got Shelbi's phone number (I didn't have the nerve to ask her for it so I asked her friend, like someone a few years younger than me might) and we would text a lot, which is initially how we got to know each other better.

As we got older, people stopped going to the camps and pressure with A-levels and University applications mounted, causing Shelbi and I to lose touch for a while. I would think about her a lot, but it wasn't until I attended a friend's wedding when I was eighteen that I saw Shelbi again. My friend (whom I also met through disabled sport) told me, a few days before the wedding, that Shelbi would be there and I remember being incredibly nervous. I didn't own any shoes that weren't trainers, so I had to make a last minute trip to town for some posh shoes. I wanted to make a good impression, and more than anything, I wanted Shelbi to like me as I liked her. I thought this could be the beginning of us being more than just friends, and it turned out to be just that. Shelbi arrived in a sophisticated black dress and, as soon as I saw her, the same feelings I'd had years ago came rushing back. It was awkward at first, having not seen each other in a long time, but it wasn't long before we were talking as we usually would. At the night party we took to the dance floor, and although that is definitely the last place I would choose to impress a girl I felt completely comfortable making a massive idiot of myself in front of Shelbi, and I have ever since.

My name is Shelbi and my Mother and Father picked my name from the film Steel Magnolias. Julia Roberts played Shelby in the film. Ironically, the girl in the film was extremely ill, as was I during my childhood. I turn 21 in the summer, and the only reason I'm looking forward to this is because I'll be able to order my favourite cocktail when I'm in America, finally! (it's a Sex on The Beach). I wouldn't say I like anything specific, but one of my greatest loves is driving (unless it's the M25 on a summery Saturday). I also love to travel and I keep tabs on more sport than most men, probably. By the time I was 19, I had driven to Germany to see Formula 1 at the Nurburgring with my Mum, and I've also driven to Belgium and Cologne. I have driven in America, and been through a drive through bank; I wasn't even aware that such a thing would exist!

My disability is always great fun, explaining to people, even family. There was a genetic mishap when my Mother was pregnant with me. I have an extremely rare bone disease called Polyostic Fibrous Displacia, to which I wasn't diagnosed until I was two years old. Because of the rarity of my disease, my parents and I were never taken seriously with 'regular' people as it was difficult to explain, and maybe sounded somewhat fake. During my childhood I was used for many medical firsts in regards to testing medicine, and my notes for my disease got to travel the world. For a period of time, I was the only female in the entirety of Europe to have both parts of the disease. To finally top this off I have a rare liver condition and scoliosis, as well as numerous pieces of metal work in my body.

The statistics of developing this are quite literally one in a million, so my boyfriend should think himself lucky! Along with the bone disease, I also have hormonal problems (more so than other females) which is the part of my disease called McCune Albright Syndrome; these are linked together. My bones break incredibly easily, and when I say this people often refer to it as brittle bone which it is not; my bones shatter or splinter when they break as oppose to cleanly, therefore it takes a lot longer for my bones to heal, along with them likely not healing properly. So when my parents agreed to let me play wheelchair sports during my teenage years, you could probably imagine their anxiety. Which I'm sure goes for any parent with a disabled child.

Throughout my life I have confused many people, not because of my good looks and incredible wit, but mainly when I park in a disabled bay and I'm not over the age of 60. I can walk short distances and I can drive a regular automatic car, how an earth can someone that uses a wheelchair be able to walk? Surely that's 'not right.' I literally see the words running through people's heads. It still completely baffles me how narrow minded some people are in the world today. One thing that I still never know how to answer is 'why are you in a wheelchair?' It's a bit like asking 'why are you standing/walking?' The look of that 'feeling sorry for you smile' is a bit old now.

I missed mundane social milestones such as birthday parties and playing kiss chase in the playground. I missed a lot of school, due to hospital appointments, broken bones and operations. My parents blame themselves for that, which I wish they wouldn't. I would have physiotherapy scheduled into my lessons at school, even though I'd miss other lessons because the lifts would be vandalised. I only finished school with three GCSE's yet I got myself onto one of the best BTEC courses I could, to get myself into university, and now I'm researching topics for my final dissertation in the coming year.

One thing my 'disability' has done for me is open up doors, as well as help me become increasingly bad at making wheelchair related jokes. However what never fails to make me laugh is when you make one in front of non wheelchair users and they're too embarrassed to laugh. Lighten up walkers, you're not perfect either.

I've wanted to push myself harder to prove people and their perception of me wrong; what they think I am or what I can do. I've done more than the average person my age, because I've put myself out there and I have wanted to experience as much as I can. One thing I am forever grateful for is the endless support of my family. I have travelled to Barcelona, Germany, Paris, Chicago and New York. Last year my parents were brave enough to let me fly to Kentucky entirely on my own, to stay with our beloved friends we met over the internet. Lauren, who also suffers with the same disease as myself, found me on the internet, and after a lot of fund-raising, determination and grit, my Mother and I went to Chicago in 2010 for a medical convention. Last year (2014) I flew out to their home and had the best summer with Lauren, Tanya (Lauren's Mum) and her family, including her dog Bella. Lauren is now one of my very, very good friends (despite the distance) and I'm sure she will be for a very long time.

Connor and I first met during a disability sports camp at Stoke Mandeville, when I was just a fourteen year old girl. The camp was the first time I had experienced anything, knowing that there were other teenagers (just like me) in a similar situation as my own; being disabled. I've not met one person who makes that the forefront of who they are, Connor more so than others which I liked straight away. It was obvious to me that Connor was shy, however once we started speaking on a more regular basis, I found out that there was a lot more to him than first meets the eye.

Thanks to Stoke Mandeville, I played Wheelchair Basketball throughout most of my teenage years, at a respectable level for my age, and this took up large amounts of my time. I also had to deal with the pressure of my BTEC and the stress of applying to university, which is when we slowly lost contact with each other. I was invited to an evening party at a friends wedding when I was 19 - it wasn't until a few days before that a mutual friend of Connor and I, had said that Connor would be there - I'm not exactly the most feminine woman in the world, but I knew when I saw Connor again I had to look amazing, I really wanted him to think I was everything that he would want. I was helped out with my newest friends I made at university, by picking out a lovely dark blue dress, perhaps slightly revealing but who cares, and some pretty shoes to match. On the night I had completely done my makeup and wore my hair down (which is very rare for me). When I entered the party and saw Connor. I could feel my cheeks warm once we started dancing, and I saw how cute he was, and I loved the feeling I got when he made me laugh, I knew that was the feeling that I would always need.

Favourite things

The first thing I noticed about Shelbi was her bright smile and her big, beautiful eyes. Even though her appearance is striking and is what drew me to her, her personality shone through straight away and is what started the connection between us. I laugh with Shelbi a lot (I adore her laugh and how infectious it is). Shelbi is very funny, and she can be silly but also sarcastic and incredibly witty, which I love. I can spend a day with Shelbi and it can be more eventful than a week with my friends. Shelbi brings out a side of me that just wants to have fun and be carefree and go and explore every corner of the world (something that we're working on together).

Once we got to really know each other I saw a lot of other brilliant qualities as well: Shelbi is honest; she says things as they are but with tact; and she is very determined, not just in sports (she can be scarily competitive), but in everything. There are very few people my age about which I could say this, but I admire Shelbi, she is a strong, independent individual. I've never had the kind of connection I feel with Shelbi with anyone else, and no matter how long those times were, when we weren't in contact, we always started talking again as if we never lost touch.

The first thing that highlighted Connor for me is his kindness. He sees good in places where I often don't; I'm a much more critical, stern person. I think this particular quality complements our relationship - we have the right balance. Most men are into football or various sports but that's my role, I am a keen fan of many American sports and Formula 1, as well as studying for a degree in Sport's Rehabilitation. However, since growing closer with Connor, I've learnt so much. Every time we're together I learn something new. His intellect and his knowledge on various different subjects really interested me. Although he's a massive gamer, has a collection of comic books taller than myself and corrects my grammar, I can't help but want to know more about the things he loves.

As our relationship evolved from friends to lovers (which took a considerable amount of time), I learnt how extremely funny, silly and adorable Connor is and that he brought out sides of me that I've not shown to anyone before. We didn't begin our voyage as a couple until I was 19, after reconnecting at our friends' wedding. From this point on I became a very fond Pogonophile (someone who likes beards) and learnt how much of a good kisser he is. I have enjoyed all of my experiences with Connor, however silly or awkward they have been. I am now an avid Star Wars fan, I appreciate a good film more and I've learnt more about comic books and superheroes than I thought I ever would, and I wouldn't have our relationship any other way.

Sex

Firstly I should point out that Shelbi and I have a healthy sex life, although it was difficult to begin with because neither of us can bend the right way. Neither of us can flex nor extend our spines, due to metalwork we have from operations, and my hips and knees are all weird. This meant that things got frustrating at times, and there were certainly points when I doubted if we'd be able to have sex. Because of this it took a lot of determination, perseverance and ingenuity (who would've known it would be easier to have sex on a sofa than a bed). On an unrelated note I'd like to thank Shelbi's landlord for choosing to have a sofa in her room. Once we'd figured out the optimum position and the best technique, it wasn't long before we began being more adventurous (make of that what you will). We now enjoy sex as any other couple would, it just took time to figure out how we would do it.

To say our disabilities have 'hindered' our sex life would be a completely idiotic thing to say; it's absolutely amazing. We took things slow at first, which I enjoyed, and then we ran into some difficulties, not because of having no desire, but because we needed the correct 'technique'. I will admit, embarrassingly, I made endless Google searches for advice and tips on how other people in similar situations have dealt with it. These ranged from 'sex with disabilties','my boyfriend and I can't have sex', 'how to have sex if you're disabled' – I will note that this doesn't make my computer history look extremely innocent. This is mainly because this isn't a regular topic that you would approach someone with, especially considering most 'normal' people do not encounter such problems. I never considered speaking to a friend about this, because it would be awkward and I'd need to explain details about Connor and myself that I would have thought they wouldn't like to know. The foreplay kept us extremely occupied during this time, although it was frustrating, and filled with endless cuddles. We then finally found a method involving a lot of will power and various pillows in awkward places, and romantically our first time was on a sofa, lol.

Did it take us a long time? Yes. Do I regret waiting or anything we did until that point? No. Would I change anything? No. Despite some tasks being difficult, such as the weekly shop, getting into pubs and clubs, or trying more adventurous sexual positions. As independent and confident individuals we've managed to travel to Cologne and Paris entirely by ourselves, whether we flew or drove to our destinations; we've now booked a holiday in Orlando for the summer; and although it may be why we met, there is one thing that has never been a major factor in our relationship - our disabilities.

James O'Driscoll is a 42 year old Personal Trainer and Actor from Kent.
He fully lost his sight at 26 and is registered blind.
He is married with a son on the way and a 23 year old daughter from a previous relationship.

James's story

Growing up - I just didn't click with school. I hated it, and often milked looking after my mum to get out of going. My Mum, unfortunately, wasn't very well when I was young. She suffered with asthma and angina, from smoking in her youth. She had stopped but it still caught up with her. Eventually, she died from cancer of the airways. It's horrible to see someone you love deteriorate like that.

At primary school, aged seven or eight, I was slightly bullied; just the nicking of sandwiches and lunch money but that's about it. I only had two fights at school: I lost one and won one!

I'd like to think that I was known at school for being a little bit cheeky but harmless. I was liked by my teachers and always got on with adults, since I have six older brothers and three older sisters. My Dad passed away when I just started secondary school so the first year of that school was horrific. I went from being in top sets to 'middle of the road' in my second year, which was exacerbated by having a lot of time off, avoiding school, and caring for my mum.

School wanted to keep me back a year because I missed so much of it but, despite everything, I did still really enjoy reading, a major secret hobby of mine. I read 'The Hobbit' when I was 12, despite hating it, and that got me really into fantasy. I remember sitting in the garden reading comics, so I was still learning even when I was off school. I can still enjoy comics even now, as they are available in graphic audio. The sci-fi/fantasy genre, and the powers that characters can have, always fascinated me. I was always more studious than sporty but there was one sport that I did connect with, however, and that was skateboarding, and something that I am only just rediscovering now.

I'm not afraid to say that I am such a massive geek. I was playing 'Dungeons and Dragons', and listening to Motown, and no-one ever knew. Now I even have Batman tattoos!

Comic books and music were my best friends at that age. I love the fact that music can teleport me back to a particular place and memory. On Sundays, I would be the first one in my family to get the stereo on. We all had a pretty eclectic taste in music: my dad liked jazz; my sister liked reggae; mum liked country and western; and my brother loved soul.

At 13 or 14, I started to appreciate girls. I realised that they didn't smell of poo and it was okay to talk to them. Since I have a decent sense of humour, I was able to make them laugh, but was quite shy with the ones I actually liked - I used to clam up and not say anything. Growing up with older brothers, porn was often found around in the house. So when I did lose my virginity, I went at it hammer and tongs, and she was making all the right noises…or so I thought. She actually just had some cramp.

At 15, I started working on the roads and loved it, with the different people, places and funny nicknames involved. Working in a physical job made my body change a lot, which I found interesting. I was making £150 whilst my friends only had pocket money, and consequently I became one of the best dressed kids in the town, with a packet of fags all to myself.

Between the ages of 15-20 I had a relationship with a girl and was 18 when I had my daughter, Stephanie. I got engaged and started saving up for a house, since I was earning really good money for my age. My girlfriend was training as a travel agent. I paid for her to go away as she was stressed but it turned out that she was seeing someone behind my back. One morning I went round to pick up Stephanie and there was no-one in. The neighbour came round to ask me why I was knocking, and it turned out that they had moved and she hadn't told me. It took me seven years to find my daughter, and I lost my sight towards the end of those seven years, so I don't know what my daughter looks like past the age of 18 months.

Losing my sight was very sudden. I went to bed on a Tuesday night and couldn't see by the Wednesday morning. I rang my boss up and told him this and he replied, 'yeah, right, you've been out on the piss.' I went to Boots for a free eye test and they sent me straight to hospital. I waited for hours to find out that I potentially had a tumour. They situated me at Kings College hospital while I waited on news about my condition and was unnerved to hear patients moaning in the night. I was diagnosed with a condition called Leber's Optic Hereditary Neuropathy causing the optic nerve to deteriorate and, much like brain cells, it cannot heal or regenerate. I often compare it being a crap Xman since it is caused by a DNA mutation. In addition to that, two years ago I also found out I have Glaucoma. [A condition affecting sight due to pressure in the eyes.] The doctors told me that the younger you are when my condition appears, the better you can adapt to it. But since I was aged 26 when I got it, my sight issues have been quite severe and I was registered blind six weeks after that first morning. I lost my job, I couldn't work and my flat was repossessed.

I grew my hair and a beard; I didn't go out; I smoked and drank too much and put on weight. But during this time I did manage to get out of a very controlling relationship. Getting rid of her was a real turning point, since I tried to kill myself twice. Her erratic behaviour, included biting herself then making it out like I'd done it. I used to go to the local shops and would get people spitting at me, since she'd told them I'd physically abused her.

One morning I woke up and all around me was just a pile of cans, fag butts and pizza.

So I went out to Argos, bought a rowing machine and did press ups every day for two and a half hours. I even rang up Quitline for smoking, just to talk to someone. I was too stupid, ashamed and stubborn to ask those around me, and who loved me, for help. My older brother has sight problems and they were all saying, 'you'll be fine,' but I wasn't fine, so I went it alone.

I developed my logical thinking and patience skills, even without being able to see, using items like Kinder egg toys and lego to piece together. It might take me a while but I will do it!

Whilst I was getting into shape, I was training at the gym once with my nephew when a guy came up to me and said, "you should be an instructor, you can really do this." Now I work as a Personal Trainer, despite avoiding sports as much as possible at school, and eventually qualified, after having nine assessments, when normally you would only have two, but they couldn't find a reason not to pass me. Before my test had even begun, they were taking photos of me shaking hands with people, so there was an awful lot of pressure. I tried in Croydon for some vacancies and, so I wouldn't be discriminated against for my blindness, I went down with my CV in person. Afterwards, I received an email from my interviewer telling me how inspired he was by what I had achieved with my disability. He had actually been made deaf after being beaten up, so related a lot to my story and what I had overcome. Three months later I was made a fitness coach at Virgin. Then less than a year later I was given an offer to be a Personal Trainer at a Bromley branch of the gym, closer to me, and have now been there four years.

I haven't always had it easy since then though. One personal trainer I work with can be a bit jealous and cocky and will actually make comments in front of clients like, "James isn't as good as me because he's blind." I trained him once and completely beat him into the ground though. I earnt his respect, even though I know I shouldn't have to, or worry what he thinks. I have worked with high profile clients and even trained professional athletes. At my last club meeting I won Employee of the Month, and the other Personal Trainer in question said, "well, it's obviously a sympathy vote." He's since been fired for not exactly being the best trainer.

My clients have always been great. I was actually the first blind person to teach a spinning class and once a deaf woman came and asked if I could assist her. I explained that I was blind and that this might be a bit of a challenge for us both. But, since being involved with Enhance, I realised I had to deal with the situation as best I could. I knew a bit of single hand sign language so me and my client kind of made up our own language for the class. I sat at the front and made simple gestures she could follow. I think she was grateful that someone had taken the time to do this with her. She sent a letter to our head office expressing her gratitude and saying how impressed she was.

Another big part of my life is acting - which I got into as a bit of a fluke. One day I heard an advert on Radio 4, from a theatre company looking for a blind actor. My brother persuaded to go, so I went, had two auditions and was offered the part. Before I knew it I was on tour with the Graeae Theatre Company for the next four years. [The Graeae Theatre champions accessibility and disabled talent in theatre and the media.] I then went and did a foundation degree in Dance and Drama at London Metropolitan University when I was 32. That's also how I met Jennie [Director of Enhance the UK] as she was my support worker there, and involved with the theatre. I never thought I would get a place on the course, but after a day's workshop and some Shakespeare improvisation, I was offered the place. My first job while at uni was working with The Crippendales, Britain's first dance troupe of all disabled strippers.

I have toured everywhere in the country with the theatre, all the way down to the arsehole end of Cornwall. It was pretty amazing. Since then, I have done bits of modelling and starred in 'Birds of a Feather,' 'Casualty' and 'Absolutely Fabulous', amongst other things. I've had lots of cool experiences, like the time I got invited to the BAFTA's by Joanna Lumley. I met loads of celebrities and had the best time.

Recently, I was flown to South Africa to perform in a tourism advert. I got the part through my agent, had two auditions and swore in my second. They did this thing where they want to film your reactions to objects, so they gave me this plant pot. It turned out to be a miniature Christmas tree. For some reason when I picked it up I went - "Mmm… Tree!" I have no idea why I said that. They said, "Keep going, explore it." So I asked if it was okay to turn it around and then went - "You'll need a really fucking small fairy for this." Then, three weeks later, I got a call from them saying that they thought I'd be great for the job.

I met my wife, Louise, through Jennie [Director and Founder of Enhance the UK.] She was her neighbour at the time and decided to set us up. Before we even met I said to Jennie, "I'm going to marry this girl." and started calling her Mrs.O. Jen thought we would be good together because she was also into sports and we are generally similarly minded. She works as an associated partner at a lettings company and deals with very high profile clients, selling and renting very expensive properties. We've been together for five years now, it's actually our anniversary very soon.

Our wedding took place in Lapland and, despite it being minus 10 degrees, I didn't even notice the cold. We had initially booked to be married in Rochester but we started getting annoyed with other people and what they wanted. One day I said, "Sod it, we should just get married in, I don't know, the north pole? We'll let Santa Claus do it." So we did. We had a whole week of huskies, saunas, ice sculptures and ice hotels. The place we stayed was very quaintly called 'Christmas Cottage.' It really is just like a great big Christmas land, with massive 30ft snowmen everywhere, and you get caught up in the whole thing. When we got there we went to see Santa straight away and he asked, "where's the kids?" And we said, "no, it's just us." So we have some great photos of us on Santa's lap.

Louise wore a tiara and a cape and looked incredible on the day; just like something from a fantasy book. She walked up in the snow to the log cabin where we were going to be married, which had these old-fashioned styled torches. It may sound corny but it was completely magical. When we were having our Christmas dinner after our wedding, a dad came over with his little girl and she asked, "are you a real princess?" And Louise replied, "well, today I might just well be."

Once, when I was away touring a play, and she was looking after my house while we were dating, she rearranged my kitchen so it was more like hers. I went to make a hot chocolate and when I put the mixture in and tried it, it wasn't sweet. After about the tenth attempt of spooning it in and still tasting nothing, I was starting to wonder what was up. Turns out she had rearranged my cutlery draw and I was using a fork instead of a spoon.

Other anecdotes concerning my sight include: accidentally locking my cat in the fridge once! (She'd jumped in whilst I was shutting the door) and another time, when I thought I was cooking oven chips and nearly burnt the house down, because it turned out I had put in runner beans instead.

In the early days of our relationship, Louise said she used to get sympathy looks from strangers, like 'aw, good for you, being with a blind guy.' If anything, I've helped her with things, like cooking and personal training. But of course, I can never drive so she will always do that for us. We've both been helping each other along, in different ways.

I'm so excited for the birth of my baby boy, my wife is now seven months pregnant, so we only have two more to go. It's crazy because you can see him moving about and everything. We've been playing him music while he's in the womb and I've been bypassing my wife's shitty taste, like S Club 7, and playing him Reef. He loves it, and you can actually see him wriggling about! He's definitely going to be a skater when he grows up!

I can admit that I can be a bit of an immature person at times, so having someone to teach and pass on all the things I love will be amazing. At least I hope he likes all the same things as me anyway, I've bought him a Batman comic already. My daughter, Stephanie, is now 23 and very successful in law and I'm extremely proud of her.

With parenting, you are always learning, and adapting, regardless of whether you have a disability or not. I have adapted in different ways throughout my whole life. I'm hopeful that my son won't experience any prejudice, having a blind parent, as his will be a completely different generation. People and their outlooks are changing and are increasingly more adapting. As my son will grow up having a blind parent, I'm confident that his attitude towards disability will be very natural.

Of course I am not finished living my life yet. As well as my expanding family, the new year has more creative work for me in the pipeline and I'll be writing collaboratively with an old client of mine on a TV project, so watch this space.

Ella Bruniges works as a freelance makeup artist and as a Communications Manager for UK Cards. Ella had a stroke when she was eight so her body has been affected by cramps, spasticity and dystonia. She is happily married.

Ella's story

When I was eight years old, I had a stroke. I was a very sporty child, but this meant that I had to relearn how to walk and talk all over again as half of my body wasn't working. My body was affected by spasticity and dystonia, and I could only effectively use my left side. I have cramp when walking, and the effects of my stroke are noticeable when I'm stressed or in any other way emotionally stimulated.

I work now as both a makeup artist and a communications officer. It felt nice working on the Undressing Disability shoot and not being looked at in a certain way. Sometimes when I work on people's make up it can be a bit awkward, when the realisation hits that I am just going to be using one hand. Make up has been really useful for me, in more ways than my career, as it can completely change a way a person looks to how they feel that day - I don't do it for anyone other than me.

At school I was quite severely bullied for being different. But I never thought of myself as having a disability as I could still ensure that I could do anything that I wanted. When I was a child, I dreamt of becoming a surgeon but of course things change. You have to live with that. I struggled with anorexia and bulimia when I was younger, as my self esteem took a beating from the cruel remarks from my peers at school. It was like I couldn't or wouldn't fit in. But now I quite like the idea of not fitting into the norm.

The spasticity effect with my stroke comes and goes depending on my mood and surroundings. If I am in any kind of 'exciting' environment, this will exacerbate it, which has at times proved difficult in dating situations. I have had botox in my arms to alleviate the symptoms but, after a year of trying for a baby, I can't have it for the time being. I have never let my disability affect the way men, or anyone, speak to me. I'm still a person who wants sex and it's been pretty hard for me, in the past, to broach the subject of my stroke on first dates.

Since mine is a relatively hidden disability it has been, at times, hard to mention. When I was younger I was definitely ashamed of my stroke. I'd say I only really grasped it about eight years ago. Before my husband, I had a few long term relationships and dates. All my partners have been understanding, as I won't stand for anybody treating me badly. Maybe that's because I don't make an issue of my disability. Once, one of my ex's made a comment about him having two hands that work and made a comment about how quick it was for him to cook and clean after a meal. I completely flew off the handle (this was when I hadn't properly accepted my stroke) thinking that he was rubbing in the fact that he could use both hands and that I was so slow. He was devastated when he realised that I'd taken it to heart. He just explained that it must be so hard on me and how proud he was of me doing things almost with one hand. It's really important to realise that people who care for you don't say things that will cause hurt, proper communication is key to making sure people are understood.

I met my husband Ross on Match.com as I wanted to settle down, and thought that going down that route would help me filter out the wheat from the chaff. He turned out to be exactly what I was looking for; it was almost love at first sight. In fact, he only lived a mile down the road from me so I was surprised that we hadn't met before. We've now been together for five years, and married for one. I'd say we had the perfect wedding for us, an intimate ceremony in a cafe where we first met.

We work really well together, and value our independence while living our lives harmoniously in parallel together. Ross works as a web developer, and both of our careers are very important to us. It's vital to us, as a couple, that we both do what we want to do, and there is no resentment between us or holding the other one back. Another thing that really helps us is Ross's laid back attitude which I think stems from him being an only child, since he hasn't had to deal with sibling rivalry or childish fighting when he was young. He tends to take things as they come, and we are very honest with each other. This is great for me because confrontation can make me very stressed, which can then make my arm curl. Together, we have a very chilled out relationship and, although Ross doesn't really have a romantic bone in his body, I like that because I prefer people to be real and not corny. And on the occasions when he does get romantic, I know that it really means something.

When speaking about my disability together, I asked him whether he's ever thought of or referred to me as 'Ella with a stroke.' He told me that, 'no, I've only ever thought of you as just Ella.' This isn't to say I have any issue asking him, or anyone else for that matter, for help if I need it regarding my disability. I am now totally comfortable asking, when in the past I may have more fiercely strived to do everything myself.

My advice to others struggling to live with or cope with their disability would be to say that it's okay to ask for help. Be honest with your best friend or any important people in your life. If you feel that there really is no-one you can turn to then there are lots of other support networks. There are friends, family, therapists, doctors to name but a few of the huge support networks that you can rely on. I think that people sometimes don't realise just how much people do care. Trying to be positive has also got me through so many scrapes. I had two recurrent miscarriages, one very recently, which was obviously a devastating experience and very isolating, but I have to be able to see the silver lining. I can eat blue cheese, rare stake, train for a 10k run.

Confidence in yourself does come with time. When I was young, I had no self esteem and went to therapy to combat this. You are unique, and that's fantastic. Now there is no way I would change my stroke. Having lived with it now for 22 years, I wish I had more consistently nurtured rather than hated my disability as part of my body.

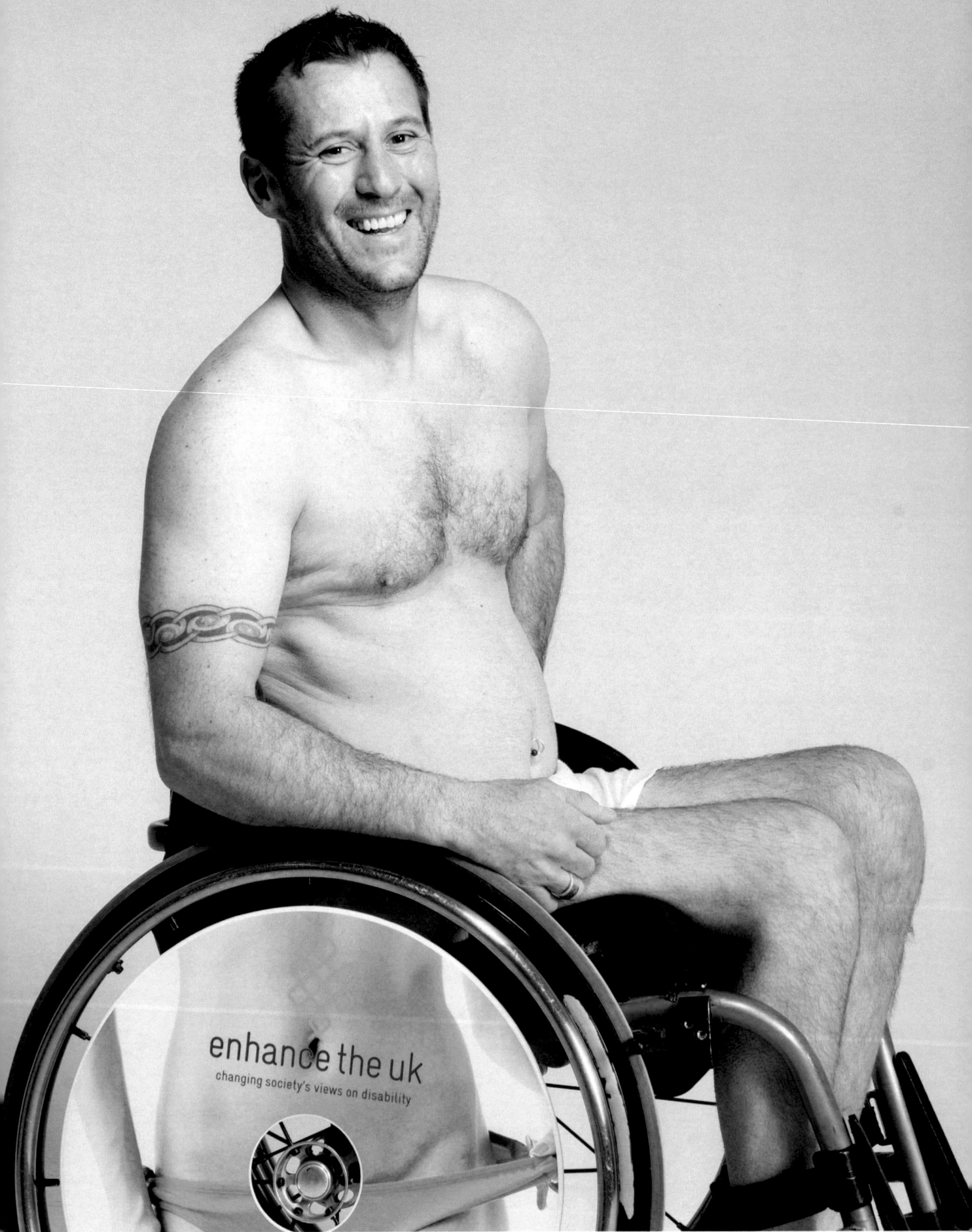

Andy Trollope is a garage owner, mechanic, water ski instructor and former semi professional motocross racer. He is a T5 paraplegic and wheelchair user after acquiring injuries in a motorcycle crash. He is also a trustee of Enhance the UK.

Andy's story

Life was good in July 2008. As I walked out of the dentist's on a sunny Thursday morning I had four things on my mind: should I ask my girlfriend of ten years Laura to marry me; the excitement of hopefully completing on our dream house on Monday; how would I perform at my first British championship race, after having my right knee reconstructed, and should I get my teeth whitened?

My name is Andy Trollope, aged 36, garage owner/ mechanic and semi professional motocross racer; yes, life was indeed GOOD. But on Sunday, 27th of July, my life was turned upside down.

While competing in the motocross British Championship event at Foxhills Motor Park on one of the hottest days of the year, and bathed in glorious sunshine, I took my place on the start line for my second race of the day.

The gate finally dropped, I released the clutch and I was off. I leapt down one of the incredibly steep hills and slowed to around 10 mph for the 180 degree corner at the bottom of the hill; I saw the big braking bumps in front of me, knowing that my suspension travel was already used up from landing after the huge leap down the hill. I braced myself for a slow trip over the handlebars, thinking, "OK, if I am quick I may be able to remount and hold my position" (not a bad position to finish the race in). After all I had been over the handlebars hundreds of times in 30 years of racing, but not many times at such a slow speed, so no worries!

That is the last thing I can remember…Apparently I was knocked out and unconscious for a while and then obviously concussed, as I have absolutely no recollection of anything after the point where I knew I was going over the bars.

I was taken to Stoke Mandeville ICU and the next few days were a bit of a blur. I had broken my T5, 6, 7 and 8 vertebrae; had bone removed from each hip to be used to reconstruct the vertebrae, and was fixed with metalwork from T5 to T8. The damage to my spinal cord was caused by splinters of bone sticking into my spinal cord, resulting in complete paralysis, with no sensation or movement from the chest down.

My parents, best friend Matt and girlfriend Laura were amazing, visiting me every single day in the ICU, making the 100 mile journey from Salisbury to Stoke Mandeville and they seemed to be there at my every waking moment. They were always by my bedside to comfort me.

During the next few days in the ICU, a regular routine was beginning to take shape. I would be woken, given a bed bath, help with eating my breakfast and getting dressed, and then a wheelchair tour to get me used to life as a wheelchair user. After a while of this regular routine things were slightly changed. My physio said "Right Andrew, we are going to do something a little different today. We are going to do a bit of physio and balance work." "Great," I thought to myself, "finally I am going to get to the gym and begin my rehab work!"

But no, I was wheeled into a side room with my parents, Laura and Matt and wheeled up to a table on which were some plastic cups of the type you would get from a vending machine. I was baffled. A physio, who was a new face to me, introduced himself as Scott (a likable Aussie guy). "Right, now that you have the basics and have been shown around the hospital, it's time we started to move things up a notch. I am going to arrange these cups in rows of four starting very close to you, and then each row will get further and further away from you. What I want you to do is work from left to right and stack the cups on top of each other a row at a time, then move onto the next row and so and so on, and let's see how far you get. Don't worry about falling, as I will be stood right behind you if you should start to lose balance, OK mate?"

Unbeknown to me, I had also suffered damage to my left shoulder as well as my back during the accident. I remember seeing Laura out of the corner of my eye, crying, and could only imagine what was going through her mind. Probably the same thing as mine - how could her big strong boyfriend of a few short weeks ago not stack up a few plastic cups, not even at arms length, in front of him? What was life going to be like for us in the future? After what seemed like an age, I managed to stack all of the rows of cups that were set out for me, although I drew no satisfaction from the simple and tedious task whatsoever.

Eventually, the move from the ICU to the rehab wards began. I was beginning to gain some independence by feeding, dressing myself, transferring from bed to chair, and getting around the hospital to my specified appointments etc. I was getting stronger by the day and putting 101% into everything I could do that would aid my rehab.

One night, I was lying in bed and thinking about getting on with life and it came to me that before my accident one major thing that was on my mind was asking Laura to marry me. So the next morning, during physio, I asked Jo if we could start my floor to chair transfers earlier rather than later (this is something that was usually one of the last things that patients were taught, as it is a very hard skill to master and in fact one that I even struggle with today). "Why?" she asked. "Well I think, actually I know, that I am going to ask Laura to marry me, and I want to be able to get down on one knee to propose and then get back in my chair."

"Oh that is exciting news!" she said, and proceeded to tell all the other physios. Now bearing in mind that 90% of the spinal physios were women, this was big news!

However, they thought the task itself would be impossible, and when I inevitably did fall out of my chair, I wouldn't be able to get back in. All this combined with the covert operations of getting me into town without Laura, to choose an engagement ring, and a trip to her parents to ask her father for his permission to ask her to marry me, made it a true mission. Thankfully, though, he said yes!

I had been in the spinal unit for four months after an initial prognosis of a nine-month stay, which was not too bad. According to Dot (who had been at Stoke Mandeville since the spinal unit was opened there) it was the fastest exit time for someone of my level, so I guess all my hard work had paid off.

When we pulled up at home, I was expecting to be staying in my neighbour's house, as to my knowledge my house was still inaccessible due to a flight of steps going up to it, and my bedroom and bathrooms being upstairs. But to my immense shock, a group of my friends had been very busy. Indeed, not only had a pathway from where I parked my car to my backdoor been built, but also a ramp up to some decking, level with the French doors, and inside there was a stair lift. Our old corner shower had been removed and a roll in shower with a shiny new shower chair was all in place. So many people had offered to help get my house ready for my return, and not one of them would take a penny for their labour. Instead, my parents and Laura had to struggle to make them take the money for materials used. On awaking the next morning, after a mammoth 13 hour sleep, and it being a Saturday, people had got wind of my return home and I was somewhat reluctantly coerced into going out for a quiet drink with a few friends. Well, when I got to the pub, I was again overwhelmed, as it seemed as if the whole of Salisbury was out and wanting to welcome me back.

I learnt quite early during my spinal unit days that there is one question everyone wants to know, and I guess this is the reason I am writing this article:

"If you are paralyzed from the chest and can feel nothing below it, can you and how do you have sex?"

Except I couldn't really answer the question about sex, as Laura and I hadn't really had sex. I mean, we had tried, whenever a spontaneous erection occurred, but quite often it would have gone down before anything could really happen.

Before I knew it, Monday came around and I was at home alone planning to get my life plan back in order. So step one, the proposal, and that meant floor to chair practice but this time, and for the first time, alone. I cannot begin to tell you about the many, many, many failed attempts and unimaginable positions that I got myself into whilst trying to do this alone, but I had to do it. After all, it would kinda take away the romance if I got on the floor, produced the ring and fell flat on my face.

I had not had the chance for a moment to arise in the last week that seemed suitable to pop the question, and seeing as it was the first week in December, I did not see any opportunity arising outdoors anywhere, so it was looking like Saturday was going to be my only option.

For some reason or another, we decided to go to the pub for a couple of pints and then just order a pizza for tea. Although Laura would not admit it, having me back was hard work. In fact, it was hard work for us both; so instead of Laura cooking, another pizza it was going to be. When we got home, we ordered the pizza and were told that as it was a busy Friday night, we would be waiting for at least an hour.

Well OK, we were in no rush and not going anywhere. As we sat in the kitchen having another beer and just chatting and chilling out, I don't know what came over me, but the way the conversation was going and just the whole evening in general, the time just seemed right. I got out of my chair, knelt on the kitchen floor and started fumbling about looking for the ring in my zipped up wheel bag. "What are you doing?" asked Laura, half laughing, half wondering whether I had fallen out of the chair or was just messing around. Anyway, out came the ring box.

I opened it and began to present towards Laura as I took the ring from it's box. Laura soon realised what I was doing and before I had even asked the question the ring was on her finger and she was saying "Yes, yes, yes!"

Then the doorbell rang, it was our pizza…great timing..! I gave Laura all that I had in my wallet, which was a fifty-pound note, and she rushed to the door, leaving me teetering, trying to remain upright on the slippery kitchen floor. After a massive hug from Laura (who had forgotten to get change from the delivery guy, so had made two guys very happy in one evening), I fell over onto the floor.

It was virtually impossible for me to get back in my chair unaided, as I was so tangled and the stone floor was slippery, but I insisted that Laura did not help. Eventually, I made it and the obligatory phone calls started to Laura's parents and friends, my parents and our friends etc. So we were engaged; there were lots of impromptu parties over the next few days as friends came to visit, but when the initial buzz had died down a bit, we began to talk about dates for the wedding.

 I suggested that we have a longer engagement as we needed time to adjust to our new life together. After all, I had only been discharged from hospital a few weeks earlier. But Laura said no, she knew what she wanted and this was it, so the planning began. I won't bore you with all the details, except to say that from my proposal in the first week of December, the date for the wedding was set for the 5th of September. Which, I have to say, is quite quick to plan any sort of wedding, but we were both extremely happy. We had a wonderful summer together (no motocross) and you know I didn't even miss it one bit. Life was again GOOD for us both.

Now I guess begins the part of my story that this is supposed to be all about - SEX.

Up until this point, Laura and I had not had penetrative sex, but if you use your imagination as with able-bodied people having sex, the penetrative part of sex can quite often be a very small part of it, but nonetheless important for both parties, but especially for me as it was more of a manliness thing. I guess just the fact of could I still perform penetrative sex after my injury, especially as I had no control or even feeling in my penis. I know that many people have asked me why it was and is so important, especially as I had no feeling in my penis nor could I ejaculate, but I could "feel" through the rest of my body in the form of, a still really unexplainable, but pleasurable kind of spasm through my stomach and my midriff.

Anyway, this is where I feel I was a little let down by the spinal unit, as Laura and I were never really offered any counseling as far as sex went, so we were kind of left to try and work it out for ourselves. So first was a visit to our GP, who I feel that I should not name as I am still under her care. I have to say that she was, and continues to be, amazing and a huge help to me both physically and mentally.

We talked things through with her and the first suggestion was to try a drug called Cialis, which you take daily and the idea is that it stays in your system and when the penis is handled or stimulated in any way should give you an erection that would last long enough for penetrative sex. This really did not work well for us, as my penis would not get hard when we wanted it to i.e. to have sex, but I could find myself at 10 am at work explaining to an elderly lady about why her hand brake was not working and what was needed to repair it etc., with a full-on erection which although I could not feel it, I knew was there as I could feel it with my hands and there was a visible lump in my trousers, which A: just felt wrong morally and B: was embarrassing should someone happen to notice it!

We tried to persevere with it, but in the end we both felt it was not for us. Then came Viagra, both Cialis and Viagra are tried and tested drugs, not just for spinal patients but for able-bodied men with erectile dysfunction. But whereas the Cialis was supposed to be taken more regularly and would stay in your system, Viagra is designed to be taken 30 or 40 minutes before sexual intercourse but again it does not guarantee an erection. It also relies on stimulation of the penis to actually work.

When at my lowest point with this particular problem for me, despite Laura's reassurances that it really didn't matter, I would quite often find myself making excuses when Laura was off to bed and obviously open to any sexual advances that I would make. Excuses like "I will just watch the end of this program or that program on TV and I will be up love". And then quite intentionally staying downstairs not really watching anything, but waiting for her to fall asleep before I would venture up to our bedroom.

So everything in our then pretty much perfect life was great except for the sex. Now I don't care who you are, sex or even just cuddles is a very important part of any relationship. As time went on, this staying up late was happening more and more, but it was something that we never really talked about. Of course, we had sex whether the Viagra worked or not, but I would be the first person to admit that our sex life was not, as you might say, a healthy one and I think Laura would also say the same.

It was by chance and at some sort of wheelie gathering, that I was to find out about the best and most reliable form of obtaining a virtual instant erection. I do not even remember how the conversation came up, but spinally injured people are incredibly open and quite often the topic of conversation when they get together turns to bladder/bowel management and sexual function. In fact this happens nearly all the time.

Anyway, I was asked, "Why are you still messing about with Viagra etc.? Have you not been offered the injections?" "Injections?" I said, very intrigued. Well, it turns out that if you can get your consultant to refer you to the sexual clinic part of the spinal unit, you can get these injections on the NHS that will give you an erection that never fails to arise within five minutes of the injection, whether your penis is being stimulated or not. Depending on how much serum you inject, you can have a permanent erection for between 1 to 2 hours and, in some cases, will work again in the morning with some stimulation of the penis. In fact, you could probably inject as much serum to give you an erection, the duration of which could be considered a medical emergency! Well this was during Saturday evening or the early hours of Sunday morning that the conversation took place.

First thing on Monday morning, I was on the phone to my spinal unit trying to get some of these amazing injections, only to find out it was not as easy as that. It couldn't clash with any other medication, and your consultant had to make sure you were getting the doses right. After pestering my consultant every day, he arranged for my first visit to see the "sex nurse" to discuss how it all worked and for my first trial. After our first meeting it was apparent that the "sex nurse" (who for the purpose of this story I will call Jane, as I think she still may well work in the same job) and I were to get on like a house on fire, even though she was a lady in her 60s and I was 36. She had been doing this a long time and had met many an eager man like me wanting to try these wonder injections.

So an injection was administered with the standard low dose, and I was sent to the spinal unit cafe and was to report back when the erection had gone down. Within minutes of Jane injecting my penis, she said "Well that appears to be working." and I looked down and there was my penis, fully erect in all its glory, probably for the first time since my injury. Trousers back up, and off I went to the café, to keep feeling for when it subsided. I must admit, I was quite self-conscious of the bulge in my trousers and having to touch myself every five minutes to feel for when it went down, but I was also grinning like the Cheshire cat.

After about 25 minutes, I felt my penis go back to its unaroused state and off I went to find Jane and let her know the time. "OK," she said when I found her (me still smiling away like an idiot), "it looks like you will not be needing a high dose, as we do not recommend that you should have an erection for any more than an hour."

After a few visits, Jane and I got the dosage right and I was shown how to administer the injections myself. Each injection comes with a tiny needle, a vial of serum and an applicator. The glass vial is put in the applicator and you open the sealed sterile needle, which you then screw to the applicator. Then, you have to press the applicator button down and squirt the serum out, until the correct amount is left in the vial for you to use. The injection site is very important for it to all work. It has to be in the base of the penis and at the side, away from any veins and definitely not into the top of the penis, as this can cause damage. After this was worked out, I was able to get the injections from my GP on repeat prescription.

But I fear it was really a little too late; although Laura and I were happy I was now beginning to force the issue of penetrative sex, but Laura and I had almost gone past that stage now and, even though we were engaged to be married, we were living together almost more like a brother and sister rather than future husband and wife.

I asked Laura several times about this, and what seemed to me to be a lack of sex life, and was she sure she still wanted to marry me for love and not out of duty, but she reassured me by saying that it was just the pressure of the wedding arrangements that was getting in the way of things.

The next thing to plan was the honeymoon. So off we went to the travel agent, telling them our budget was £7,000 and the only real stipulations were that we wanted somewhere hot, and the most important thing of all was that I could get around and go to any poolside bars of the complex unaided, as it was pretty certain that all Laura would want to be doing during the day was sunning herself, whereas I would get easily bored doing this. I would not want to have to drag Laura with me every time I wanted a beer or to go back to the room. Well, we were in luck as we were told that there was a recently refurbished hotel complex with no steps anywhere, and easy access to everywhere, on the Island of Mauritius. It sounded perfect, so it was booked and that was one less thing for us to worry about.

I will fast-forward a bit to the wedding. It was, and still is, one of the best days of my life to date. I can still remember the gasps of shock and the look in Laura's face when, after her Father had walked her down the aisle and as we were about to say our vows, I flicked the levers on my new wheelchair which actually was, unbeknown to anyone except my parents and the best man (my best friend Matt), a standing chair and I was standing bolt upright, and looking directly into Laura's eyes, as we said our wedding vows before God.

An hour later we left the church as husband and wife. After the photos, confetti and all the other stuff that goes on outside the church, we were driven the short distance to the reception venue. Speeches were delivered, the cake was cut and we had our first dance together as husband and wife.

Then began what I can only describe as probably the best party I have ever been to. It was not until day was breaking and the last guests had left that Laura and I were able to really see each other, as each of us was in such demand by various people throughout the evening. Totally shattered, the last thing on either of our minds was sex and consummating the marriage. There was still the honeymoon to come…

The first thing we were greeted with in this "no steps anywhere in the complex" was a huge grand marble set of steps up to the reception. Laura and I just looked at each other, both travel weary from the long flight, but the manager came rushing out "Mr. Trollope we have a disabled ramp just to the side for you to go up to the main reception, welcome, welcome! "

We checked in and were shown to our "disabled friendly room". Problem Number one, the door threshold was so high that I could not enter room unaided. Problem Number two, I could not even enter the toilet as the doorway was so narrow. Problem Number three, a four inch threshold to enter the shower room.

Sohe hotel staff showed us what seemed to be endless room after room to try and support my needs; in the end they finally showed us their top room, which was a mini beach-front studio-type room, but the threshold was still too high and the toilet doorway was enough for me to jam my wheelchair in the doorway and make a 180 degree transfer on to the toilet. The hotel manager and staff (who were great, very helpful and I think a bit embarrassed by the whole thing) said that this was the best they could offer us and was, in fact, the "best suite that the hotel had to offer". Too tired to argue anymore and by this time thoroughly pissed off, we said we would accept this "mini villa" as we just wanted to sleep.

So we went to sleep after our first argument of many during that honeymoon. I think it went something along the lines of me saying "I expected more than this for seven f***ing grand!" and Laura retorting with the line of "Well, if you had taken more interest instead of working every time I went to the travel agent, perhaps it would have been different!" And so on that note, on the first night of our honeymoon we went to bed, each picking a side of the enormous bed and went to sleep.

The honeymoon did not go as planned and although we had a nice time, it wasn't the great time a honeymoon should be. We had great days and did great things, but it was marred by arguments about the problems caused by the inaccessibility of the whole place and just lots of petty arguments that you would not expect two people in love, and on the supposed honeymoon of a lifetime, to have.

After coming back to the UK and settling into our new lives as husband and wife, things actually seemed a bit better than when we were on honeymoon. We were getting along better, with fewer arguments, but still no sex. I am sure we must have both tried to initiate lovemaking at some stage, but for one reason or another it just did not happen. I was just trying to be patient with Laura and maybe she had just realized the full implications of being married to a paraplegic, or maybe I had changed, but I didn't feel as though I had. Maybe that was part of the problem, I don't know. But whatever the reason, on the 11th of November I got a phone call from Laura saying that she had packed up most of her things, was moving back to her parents in Basingstoke and she would arrange to pick up the rest of her stuff at a later date. I raced home as soon as I could, but she was gone and was not answering her phone to me. We met up several times to talk, the first time being less than a week after she moved out. I noticed that she was not wearing her engagement or wedding rings and she was adamant that she was not coming back, as it was all too much for her to take. During many other meetings, I made promises of trying to change, that we could work it out, but there lay the problem. She could not give me any reason for leaving, other than to say that she was not happy. It was agreed that, as we had a large house, she could leave her stuff in it, as it would not all fit at her parents' home. So I was left alone at home, finding myself waking up, staring at an empty bottle of Jameson's on many an early morning, quite often too drunk to go to work. Or even waking up on the sofa, halfway through our wedding DVD, and trying to work out how we had got from that happy day, not so long ago, to here - another thoroughly miserable day. After a few weeks, with the help of my amazing family and friends, I got myself together enough to be not hitting the whiskey bottle every night and I was back at work, still making contact with Laura and still getting the same answer that she was definitely not coming back to me.

Christmas was fast approaching and I felt, and other people agreed with me, that I needed to get away for a change of scenery. I had no idea where I was going to go or indeed who with. After a long chat with one of my close friends on Facebook, who had moved to the island of Koh Samui in Thailand several years earlier and another friend who had been living in Bangkok for over ten years, I decided that Thailand was the place for me. Laura and I had visited Darryl on Koh Samui some years earlier and had had a great holiday. So immediately after that conversation, I was online, booking my ticket and two days later I arrived on the tiny Island of Koh Samui. My ticket was open ended and, although I planned on staying for about six weeks, my stay was nearer to three months.

To begin with, I was content with lying by the pool all day with the occasional swim and a few beers and, as often happens in Thailand, the memories of life, work, pressure and to some point even Laura were beginning to fade. Messages were beginning to come through to me that Laura and her friend had also decided to go to Thailand, so I guess it must work for everyone?

From day one, Darryl had been trying to get me to go out with him and meet some girls but, as I kept protesting, a woman was the last thing on my mind. But one day when he asked me, I think as much to my surprise as his, I just said "Yeah, ok". We arranged to meet later that evening at around 10.30pm, as the bars do not really get going until around then. This was the first time that I had really been outside of my hotel complex at night, and my jaw just hit the floor. The small open-fronted bars were just overflowing with some of the most beautiful women I had ever seen.

After about five minutes, we went down one of the many side streets and into a small open fronted bar and ordered a drink. There were not many men in this bar, but it was overrun with women, every one of which knew Darryl and, I suspect, had slept with him. After all, he had been living there for over 5 years. While we were drinking our Red Bull and vodkas, Darryl said to me "So then mate, any of these take your fancy? You can have any of them and the prices are good!" This was my first introduction to prostitution in real life, and it did not sit well with me. Were these girls being forced into it? Were their families being threatened? All these thoughts were going through my head, as I always knew that 99% of men traveling to Thailand were going because of its booming sex trade. But when you are in that situation for the first time, well for me anyway, it felt wrong. I questioned Darryl on this and he explained that some did it to save money to go to college, some did it voluntarily to send money back to their poorer families and some just did it because they liked it and liked the money, so there was no need to feel guilty about it. "Just get on and have some fun, that's what you're here for isn't it?" "Well no, not really." I said (but I guess it was always in the back of my mind).

Darryl explained the rules; so if you liked someone and they agreed to go with you, you first had to pay their 'Bar Fine' which is basically a payment to the bar owner/ manager, or Mama San as they were also called. You then had to first agree whether you wanted "short time", which was my understanding of prostitution, where you and she would go off for an hour to have sex, a blow job or whatever it was you had agreed. Then she would be back at the bar after going for a shower etc. Well, this was obviously out of the question for me, as it could take nearly the allotted time for me to get dressed and undressed, let alone do anything! So it would appear that "long time" was my only option, which again you would agree with the girl that she would go with you (normally to your hotel room) and stay the night. But of course, she would have to agree this with the Mama San that she could leave for the rest of the night and the bar fine would be higher as would the payment to the girl (which you should always agree before you leave the bar). This appealed to me much more, also as it did not seem so seedy.

One night, we were in a bar that we had frequented a few times and there was one girl in particular that I would spend time talking with. It wasn't just bar talk, but really talking about her family and my disaster of a marriage and I genuinely liked her. So, the deals were done and we went off and had a few drinks, then went back to my studio in the complex. We talked for a bit and then had the most mind-blowing sex of my life. We went to breakfast the next day and there was no awkwardness between us. After breakfast we went back to my room and I paid her. Then we had yet more sex (for free). Her name was Som and after sex and the obligatory shower for us both, she offered to show me around the Island. So I had a beer, doubting if I would see her again that day. But true to her word, she came back in an open-topped Suzuki jeep. I transferred into the passenger seat and she put my wheelchair in the back and off we went. She took me to see some of the most breathtaking sights I have ever seen; waterfalls, Buddhist temples and beautiful small secluded beaches, and some great tiny roadside eating places. She also explained that the places we had been to were not on any tourist maps and, in the main, only Thai people knew about them.

Well, a perfect day was coming to an end, or so I thought. When I asked her what time she had to go back to work, "She said 8 o'clock unless you want me to stay with you tonight again?" Still a little green about all this, I said "Well, what do I owe you for today?" "Nothing," she said, "Today was my time to spend how I wanted and I wanted to spend it with you!"

So we spent the next night and day together, and the next and the next. In total, we spent the next 3 weeks together, sometimes going out in the day, sometimes playing around in and out of the hotel pool, sometimes going out to other bars to meet her friends and sometimes just staying in my studio, having sex all day and all night.

Darryl gave me a bit of a talking to and said "What are you doing man? I have seen this time after time; blokes come to Thailand and meet one girl, then stay with them the whole time! There are literally thousands of girls out there! Go find another one, she's only using you because you are easy money and she doesn't have to go back to work and get to sleep with some old or fat bloke! Wait till she tells you how much you owe her, she will have ripped you right off!" I could see his point, as Som and I had become nearly inseparable. She was even taking my washing to the laundry for me and collecting it, pairing socks, folding t shirts and putting them away or hanging them up.

Andy's story

So I decided to end our arrangement and take Darryl's advice to go and have a look around and find someone else. I told her one morning thinking she may be upset, but she simply said "I knew this was coming, but it's fine. When I met you, I could see only sadness in your eyes, but now I can see happiness. It's time for you to go out and meet new girls, this is good for you!" We went back to my room to work out the finances and it was only when she had gone that I realized she had not charged me anything for the days and only charged me for two weeks, not three, of the nights. So, confidence restored, Darryl and I were hitting the bars every night and I guess I just got used to taking home a different girl every night. Sometimes the sex was OK, sometimes it was good and sometimes it was mind-blowing! Not one of these girls was ever put off by my catheter and leg-bag. Some even asked what it was for, and some even insisted on emptying it for me so I did not have to get up to do it myself. Som and I even had a few more interactions, when the occasion arose, and she would never be jealous, but just say, "I see you sleep with many Thai women, it's good for you!" And so that was my life, either sunning myself by the pool or going out and having amazing sex every night. It's understandable why so many men holiday in Thailand! I even had my first ever threesome whilst I was there!

Soon, however, it was time to go home. Once back in the UK, normal life resumed but without Laura. I returned to work and quickly got back into the swing of things in general. One thing though was different about me. I found that I was full of confidence with life in general, but especially around and in the presence of women. On a night out, I was no longer the guy sat in the background, I was on the dance floor in my wheelchair, dancing with women who, up until that point were complete strangers. I was asking them if they wanted a drink or somewhere to sit, i.e. on my lap, and just flirting in general. It was around this time that I had a phone call from Laura that blew me away. We had had no contact since before we both went to Thailand, as neither of us were in a hurry to actually start divorce proceedings and she knew that her stuff was safe at home. She called me up out of the blue saying that she was now having second thoughts about our marriage and had said her vows before God and intended to keep them, so would I consider marriage guidance counseling? Well, I had been living a single man's life for quite a while now and was enjoying it, or was I really?

After a few phone calls and face-to-face meetings with Laura, I agreed and she had found a counselor in Salisbury that could see us once a week in a few weeks' time. Laura had offered to pay for the sessions and so the lines of communications were again open between us, talking on the phone once or twice a week before our sessions actually began.

The big day arrived and we had our first of the six sessions that Laura had booked. In all honesty, I think that we were closer to getting back together before we started having counseling, as all that happened was that we were virtually at each other's throats at the end of each session, whereas when we were just talking on the phone we actually talked. But in the counseling sessions, we were forced to face the actual problems we had with each other, and what we disliked about each other. I guess this is what is supposed to happen, maybe to actually bring those problems to the surface and try to resolve them. The trouble was that they seemed irresolvable. At the last of our scheduled six sessions, the counselor said to me "Andrew, I am getting the distinct feeling that you don't want to get back with Laura at all."

I paused for a long time, and I think I was just thinking of Thailand and the past few months living as a single man and not of the ten years of relative happiness that Laura and I had spent together. After the long pause I simply said, "No, I don't think I do."

Laura is now remarried and has two children. We do keep in contact, but to a bare minimum. She helped me fill in some of the gaps in this story. As for relationships and sexual encounters since then, there have been multiple one night stands. Not that I am proud of them, but they happened, so I may as well admit them. As I cannot ejaculate and have no feeling in my penis, I am not like other men, or indeed myself prior to my accident, and I don't just want to get it inside someone as soon as I can.

I don't just have sex, I make love and as I can't come myself, I get most of my enjoyment from the kissing and the cuddling side of things. My chest and nipples are extremely sensitive and I get off by getting my partner off as many times as possible. In fact, and only then, will I suggest (unless, of course, they should suggest it before me) getting my penis erect by either the use of a Viagra tablet or two (very unreliable after a lot of alcohol), or the 100%-efficient method of the injections, that is unless you are so drunk that you miss your penis and inject your finger. You end up with a limp penis and a finger that you cannot bend for a couple of hours. Trust me… I know!

You may laugh, but it was my misuse of those oh so wonderful injections, that left me with an erection for so long that I can no longer achieve one regardless of what injections I try. If I had not been put forward by my amazing urology consultant for pioneering surgery, I would never have been able to have penetrative sex again. I have had implants inserted into my penis and a small finger pump in my scrotum. This allows me or my partner to pump up and let down my penis as and when we wish. So please, do heed the warnings, they really are true!

So let's fast forward to today. Well, I am in a relationship and we have a very healthy sex life - sometimes using my pump up penis, sometimes not. We are in the very early stages of an IVF program and life is again GOOD for me. So it would appear that my life has gone full circle.

My advice to anyone who has a spinal cord injury is that it is a shitty thing to happen,

I won't lie to you. You will have good days and bad. You have to make the choice between giving up and fighting.

If you keep on fighting like I have, then it's still a shitty thing to deal with, but one thing I will promise you IT DOES GET BETTER. Who knows, you may end up as happy as me. I certainly hope so.

Thank you for reading.

Andy

T's story

There was this girl at university. I first saw her acting in a play, and thought she was very attractive indeed. I was less than prepared when, after the play, she came over to the bar I was sitting at and offered to buy me a drink. My friends left us to it, we were all alone. What a romantic opportunity I had in front of me…I was 19 at the time, hugely insecure, and still thinking about the pretty cruel bullying I had experienced at school. This girl opposite me, as gorgeous as she was, just made me freeze. I had the opportunity to buy her a drink, possibly go on dates and more, but I was so terrified that she'd see me walking funny, see my disability, that she wouldn't want me. After a while of awkward silence, I just said I had to go, got up and left.

I'm T, 34. I grew up in Essex and have cerebral palsy (predominantly in my legs) and dyspraxia, which affects the rate that I absorb and process information. Who'd have thought that the guy who once sat like a rabbit in the headlights in front of a girl who was blatantly into him now works as an actor and dancer, busting his moves for a company that work with disabled artists, to create and promote integrated drama and dance works?! I'd always been interested in drama, right from doing it at school, and I knew that I wanted to follow that path through university, and eventually make it my career… I just didn't know if my disability and lack of self-belief would let me. I went to a mainstream school that was enjoyable on the whole. I had the support of the SEN unit, although I rarely used it (apart from getting a swanky computer to help with my reading rates, a note taker to write for me whilst I listened, and a support worker making sure I didn't spill acid all over myself in science lessons!) I also had a great circle of close friends at school. I was however, badly bullied, and went off to university with little confidence about myself, especially my appearance.

It was in my mid 20s that I finally stopped worrying too much about what people thought of me and my funny walk, and started doing things that would promote my own personal growth. I went on assertiveness courses, started practicing meditation, and took sign language classes as part of my degree (although this didn't really help with family harmony when I ended up calling my Dad pregnant…) I also used the drama and dance that I had always loved as my own healing process. I slowly started to appreciate the wonders of my own body and what it could do, and studied movement to help me understand that my physicality was and is unique. It is special and should be celebrated. These realisations encouraged me to change my perception of myself. I finally realised that it was my perception that had created a barrier for me over so many years, and once I built up my confidence, no barrier was really there at all.

Before the age of 28, I had been concentrating on just getting through life; girls weren't even on the radar. Even if they were, I couldn't face up to the possible rejection if I asked them out. But after getting into touch with my body and abilities, I had the confidence to speak to women, and was comfortable knowing that the more I liked myself; the more likely I was to attract somebody who liked me back. I still believe this now, and know that if someone is the kind of partner I'd like, then they're going to be positive and kind and offer support around my disability. I wasn't, and still wouldn't be, interested in someone who offered negative comments. That is one thing about having a disability, it does act as a filter for finding the good in people.

I knew I had found a good person when I met H just after my 28th Birthday. She was compassionate, sweet and beautiful, inside and out. We had common interests, a love of the Arts, and both wanted to challenge ourselves and seek adventure. I thought to myself, "I'm definitely going to fall for her!" But here's the surprise to the story. I didn't, not fully, not like she did for me. I was so attracted to her, but it was almost a constant fancying, a half-way zone, never quite leading to the big L word. I wanted her, but knew it wasn't going to be forever. We ended our relationship after about 6 months, but it ended nicely which makes me happy. She's just got married actually, and I do feel the lonely pang of what could've been, but we've both moved on to new life stages now, I guess. H really helped me to figure out who I am and what I'm about. I'll always be grateful to her for that. I became much more confident about my body when I was with her, and we both felt comfortable enough to sit down and talk about sex, our likes and dislikes, and any challenges it might bring up before we had a sexual relationship. The physical side of things was great, and I'll probably always be a bit attracted to H because of what we experienced together.

After we broke up, I went travelling, found the confidence to use dating sites, and I'm now getting myself 'out there' to increase my chances of finding someone new. I feel ready for a new relationship and want it to have the same warmth, openness and honesty that I shared with H. I'd like to be with someone who enjoys and searches for spontaneous and adventurous things, someone who likes to challenge themselves. On a personal level, I would also trust my instincts more, and not freeze like I did with the attractive girl at university.

When something is right, you just know, and I never want another 'what if' experience. But it is also important that I am gentle with myself; what's the point in beating ourselves up over missed chances and spilt milk? I'm now ready to take a chance, and cannot wait to see what new opportunities, in love and elsewhere, are around the corner for me.

Love, T

Andy and Mitchell's story

My name is Andi, I'm a 30 year old female from Memphis, TN and when I was 26 I met a gentleman who is now my fiancé. Mitchell is unlike anyone I had ever met in my life. The first time I saw him in person, I immediately felt the most genuine sense of wellbeing; a happiness came over me, because at that moment I knew that we were going to be life long friends. He is the most caring, understanding, happy and genuine individual I have ever met.

Mitchell was born with a genetic condition known as osteogenesis imperfecta which causes your bones to become very brittle and break easily. He has type three OI which causes more breaks and stunted growth than other types, and has experienced breaking over 200 bones, 22 surgeries, and has cardiac arrested twice. He is a miracle that I can't explain. I believe we were always meant to meet.

Here is a little background about the two of us: we both grew up in the same subdivision as kids/teens and attended the same high school (half of it during the same time, I am two years older). His father was in the navy and stationed in the Jacksonville Florida area. My dad was also in the navy and we were stationed there as well. We had never met or knew/spoke of the other until he was 23 and I was 26. He had never been in a real serious relationship before meeting me, and I had just ended a six-year relationship. I was acquainted with his brother through mutual friends of ours. We had only hung out once, that I remember, and that was for a homecoming dance that we attended with our mutual friends. We both graduated high school and during all this time I never knew of Mitchell.

One night after reconnecting through Facebook, his brother and I decided to hang out and have a drink. During a conversation at the bar, trying to recall the name of one of Jack White's bands (it was The Dead Weather by the way) he called his brother, Mitchell, as he would surely know. Mitchell had just been to a Dead Weather concert. We found out that we shared similarities in music taste after I told him I attended a White Stripes concert, and he told me he had missed that one and really wanted to see it. By the way, all this music convo is occurring after commandeering the phone from the brother because Mitchell and I both were getting tired of the middle man. Later that night, Mitchell asked if it was ok to get my number. It wasn't long after, I received a text from him and so began a month long of talking.

When I finally worked up the courage to hang out with him, I picked him up from school. He was attending an art school for a degree in sequential narrative and had already obtained a degree in graphic design. Needless to say, Mitchell is an artist. I'm a nurse. I guess being a nurse made caring for Mitchell easier (as he does not walk.) Although he cannot walk he has accomplished so much and always strives to bring happiness to other people's lives. Mitchell helped me when I became sick with Graves disease (an autoimmune thyroid condition) and always supported me and pushed me to heal and be happy.

I moved in with Mitchell who was living with his mother at the time, and we lived there together for two years. Mitchell graduated and has being doing lots of art/work since graduating. I found a job I love. Things always continue to work out. We are each other's soul-mates and connect spiritually, in ways I never thought were possible. The luckiest day in my life was when I decided to drink a beer with an old friend, on a Tuesday.

Mitchell's Story.
We get very strange looks from people. If Andi is wearing scrubs they definitely think she's just my nurse. But if she's in normal clothes, people look at us as if she's my mom or something. So we just make them feel very uncomfortable by making out!

I know when we first met, people were asking if she was using me. People were asking her what she saw in me. Most people make a lot of assumptions about people in wheelchairs, or people who are very short. They assume I can't function or that I'm too small to function, when the reality is the exact opposite. When I graduated art school I did a full scale full body nude photo/X-ray of myself. Called "Just Skin & Bones" which deals with how people stare at others that aren't perfect.

To be honest, sex is very important to our relationship. We personally believe sex is important in any relationship. Andi was the first girl I ever slept with, so I was very nervous, but also couldn't wait. Andi searched the Internet on "how to have sex with someone with brittle bones." Google doesn't answer that by the way. We happened to meet right before my birthday. And when it came around, she showed up at my house and it felt like something out of a movie. She had a vinyl of The Deftones, White Pony (because I'm a vinyl nerd). So she stripped and carefully got on top of me. It was the best birthday I had ever had. Normally people's first time ends fairly quickly. But not me. I'd say if I was nervous, but we had sex for four hours the first day.

Then, four more hours the next time, until I finally relieved myself. Another time we stopped right in the middle and decided to switch positions. When we did she moved wrong and kicked my toe with her knee, breaking it. Sex for us can be interesting. It didn't take very long to figure out the most comfortable position. As far as kids go we are both able to conceive but neither of us want to. With us both having illnesses, we feel it's just cruel to bring a baby into this world knowing it's going to be sick. If we ever really want a kid then we will adopt a child.

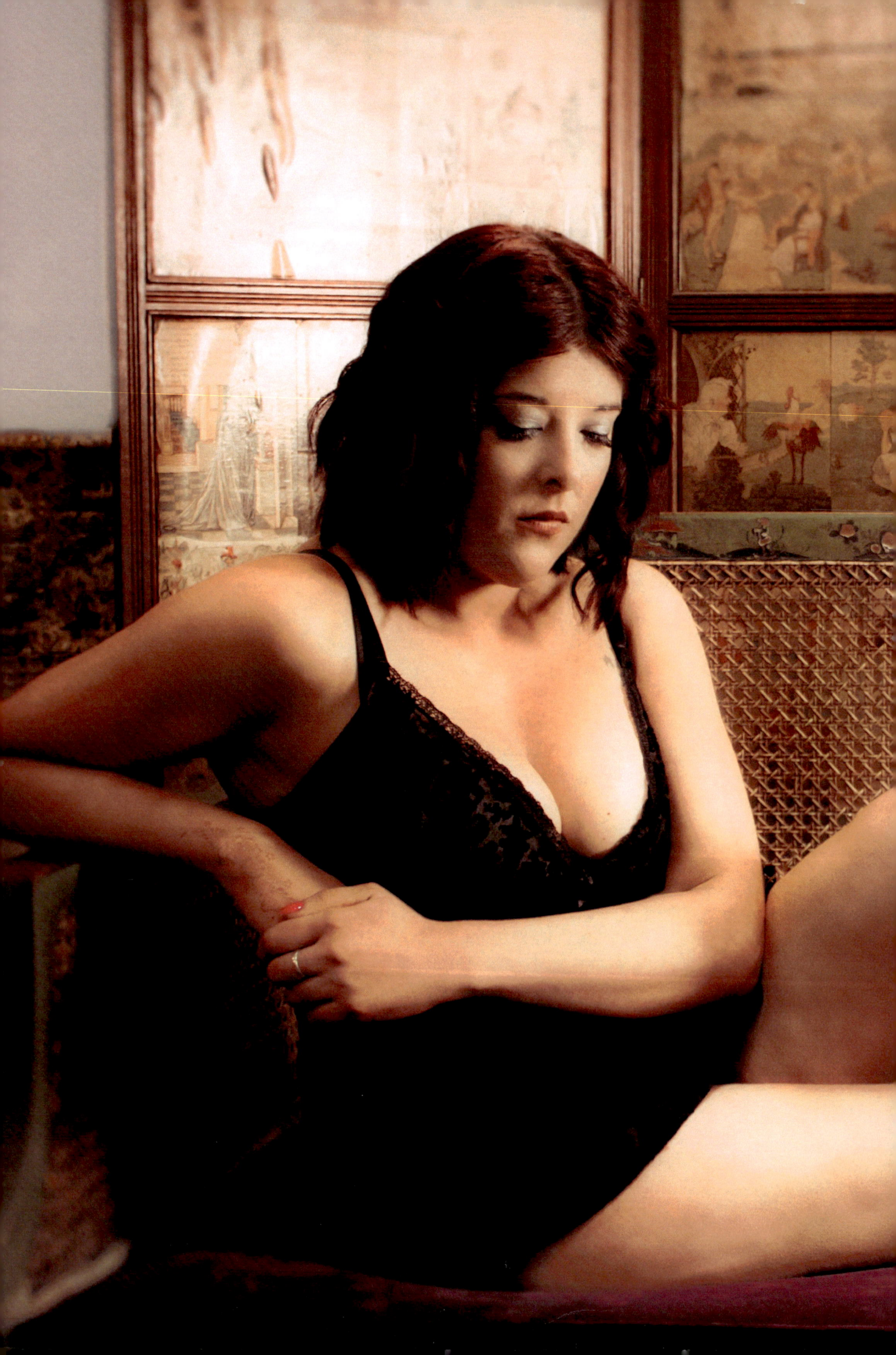

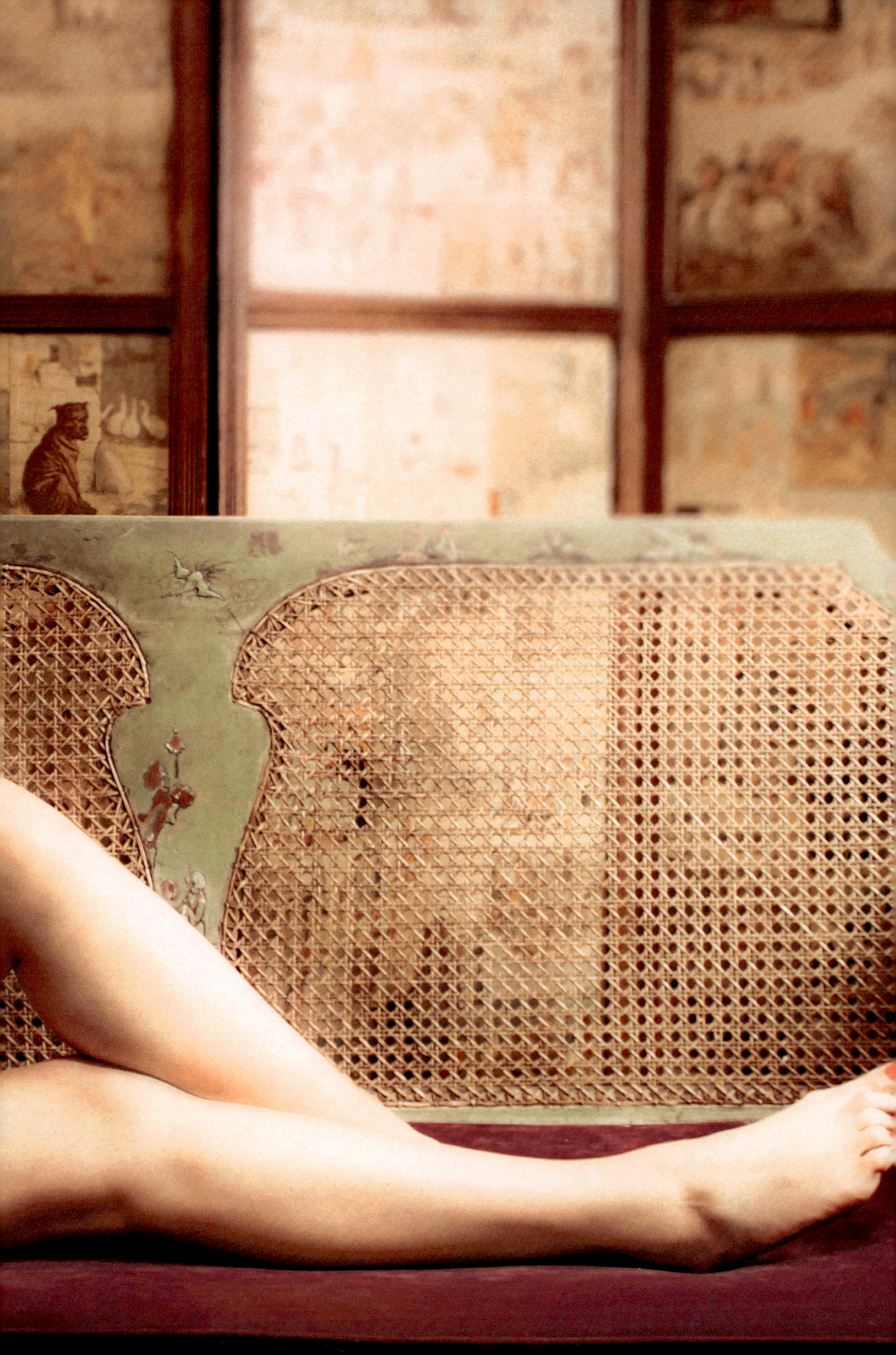

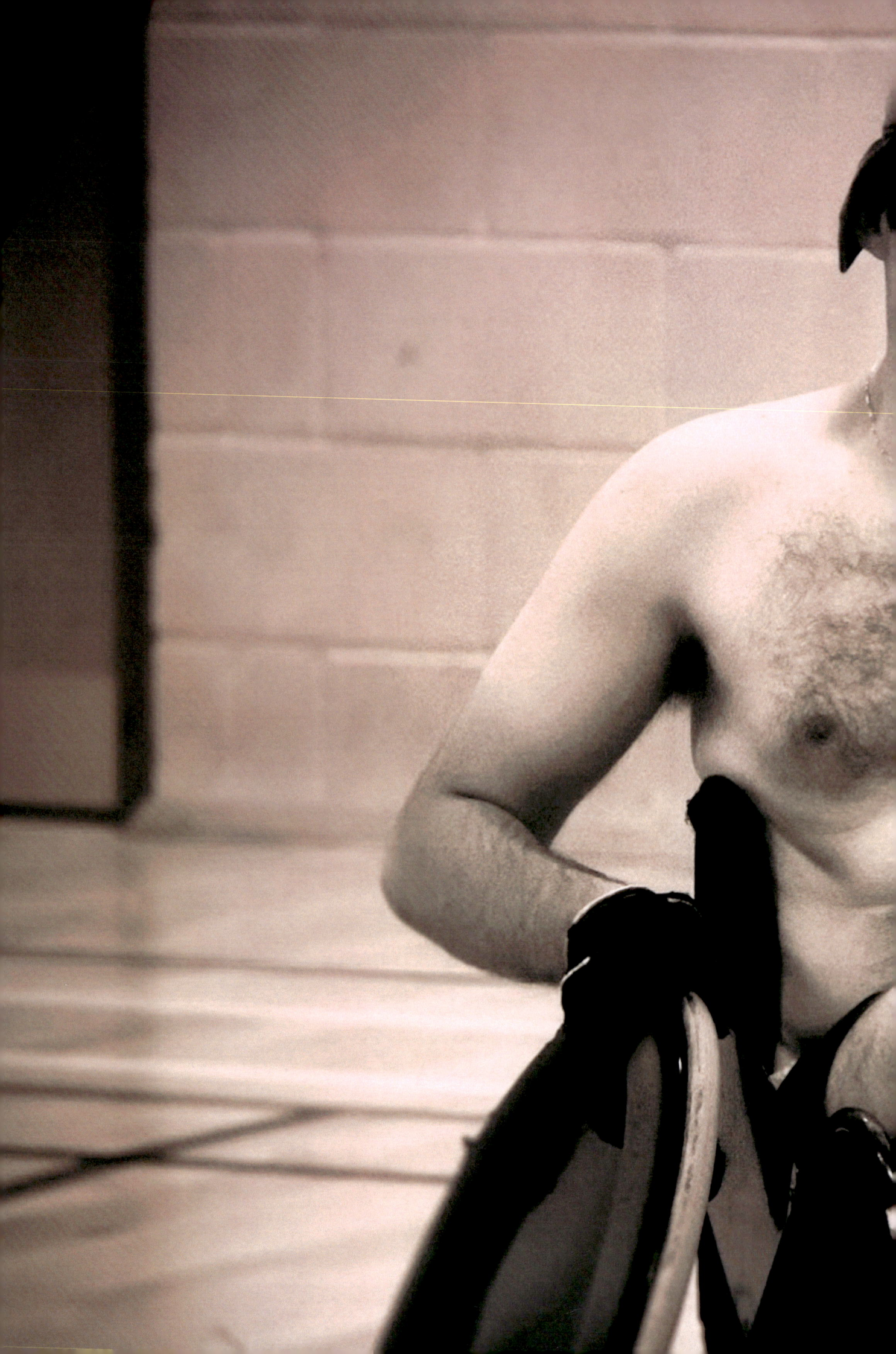

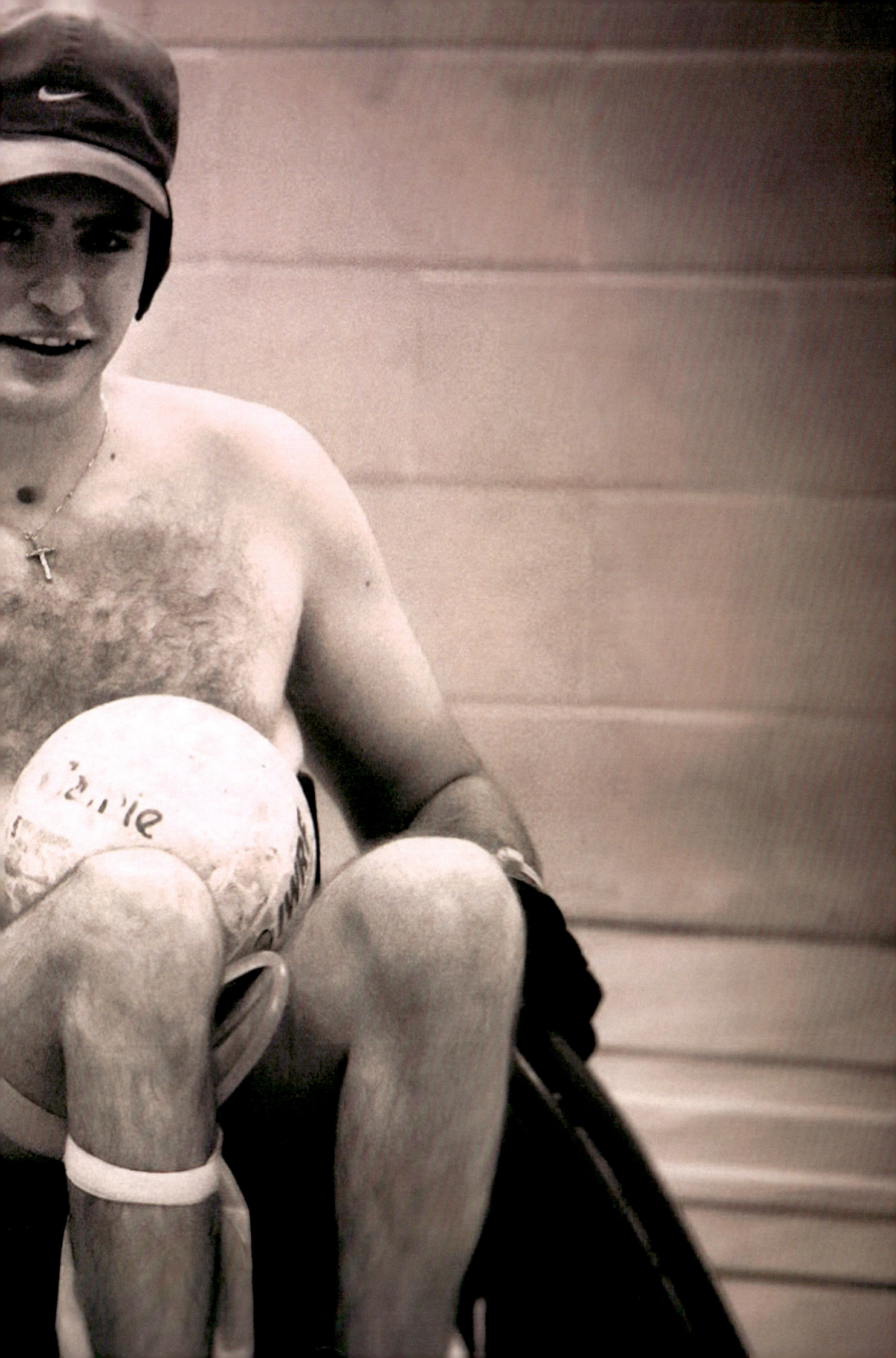

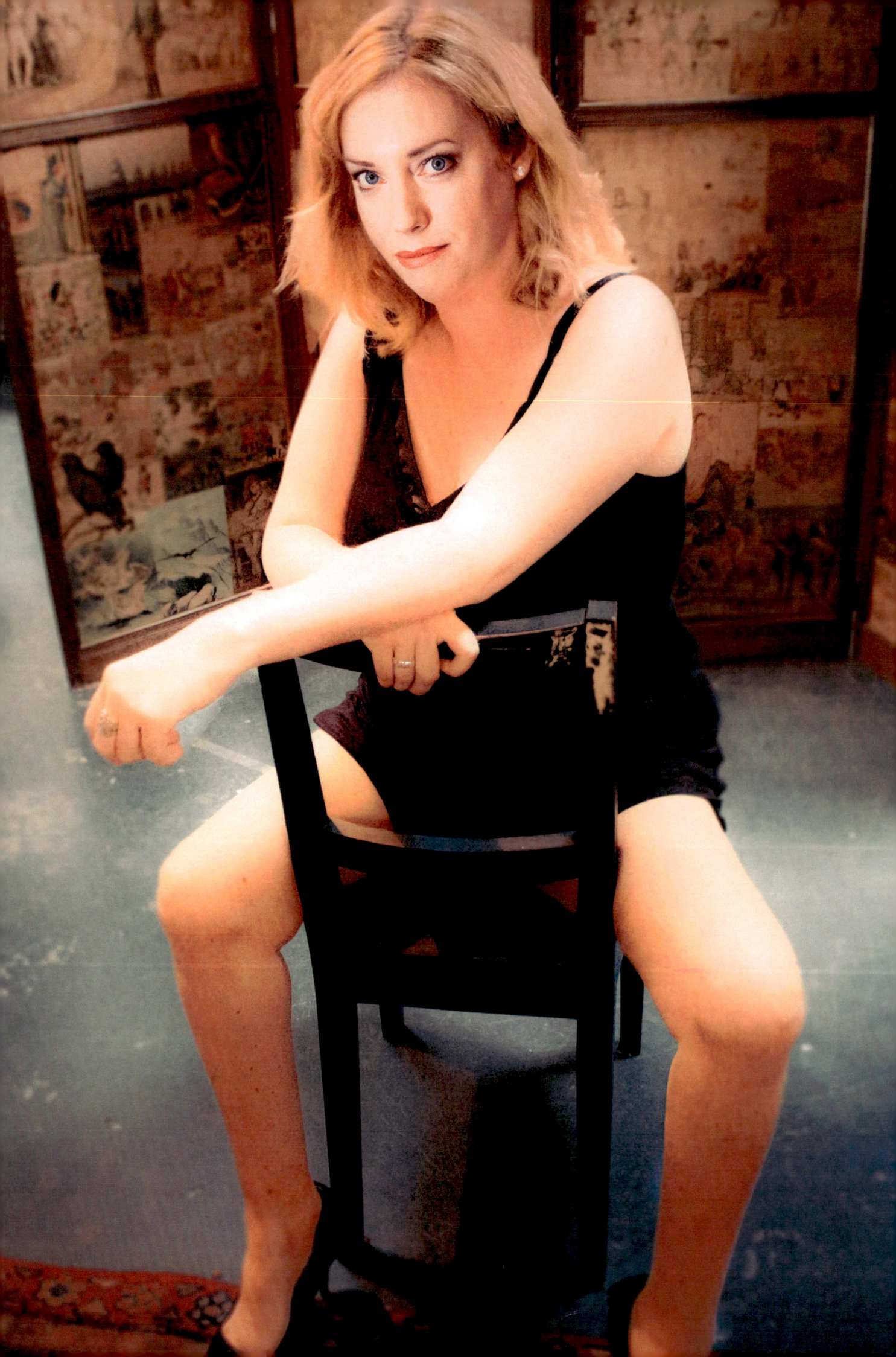

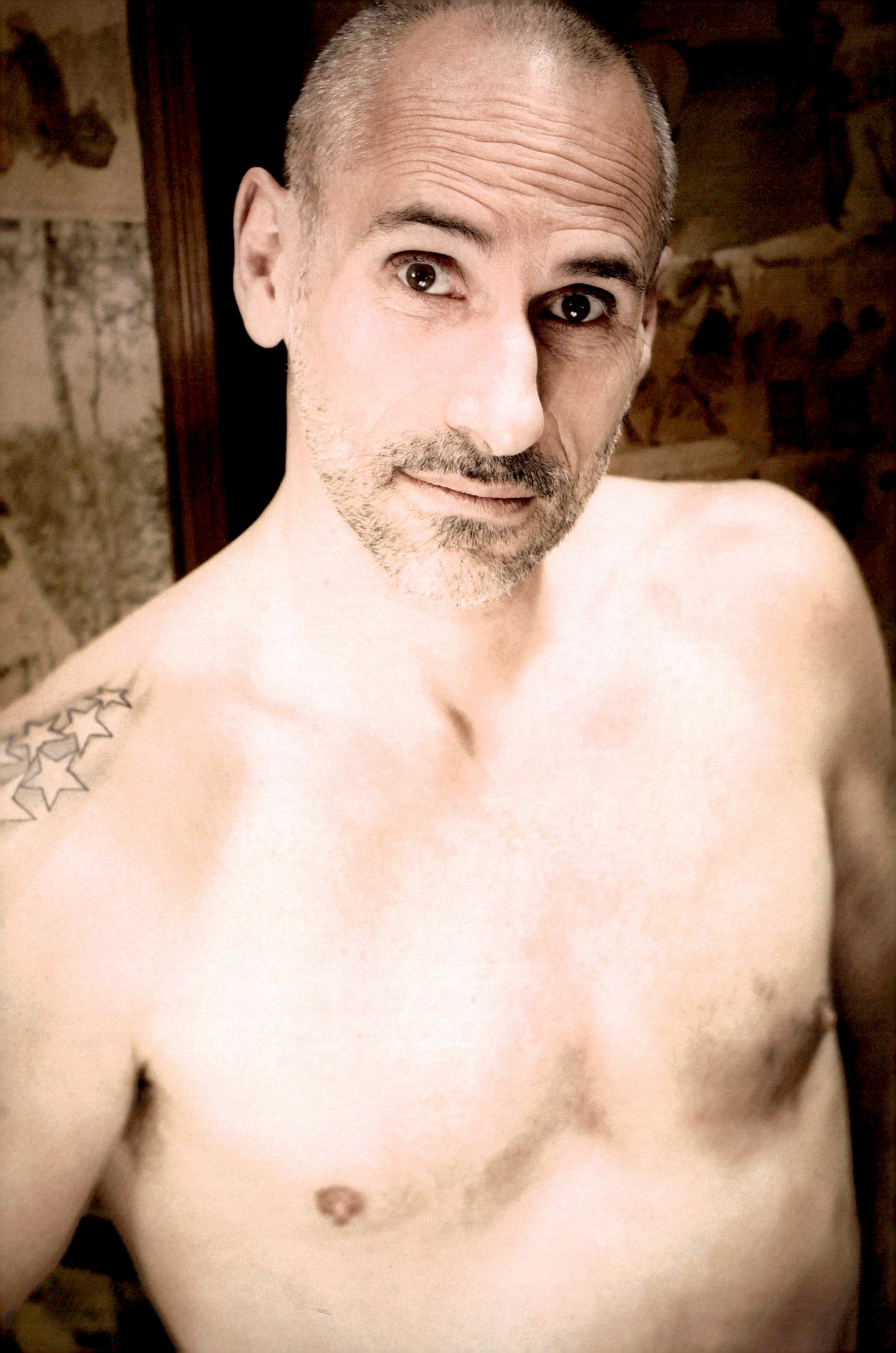

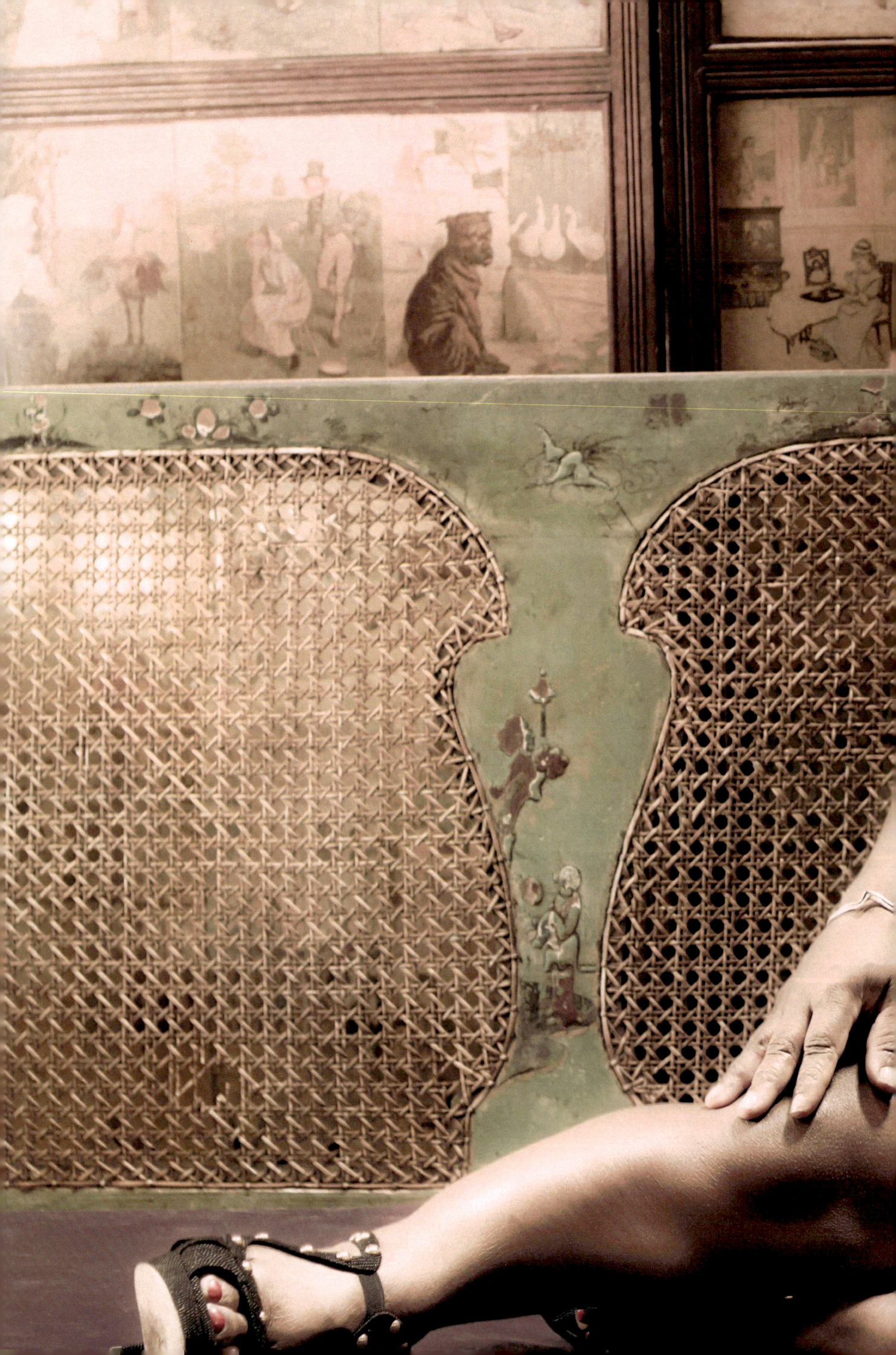

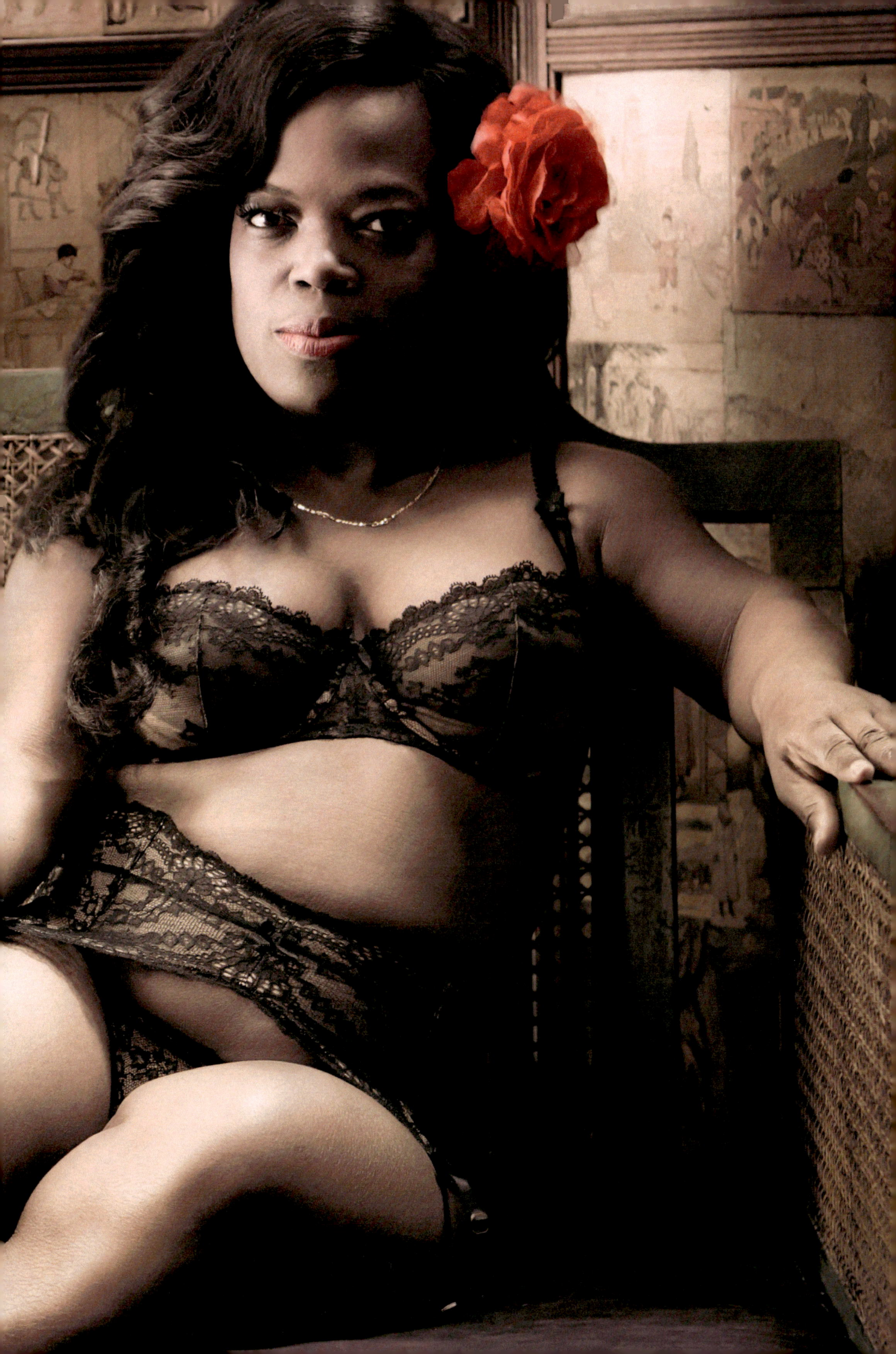

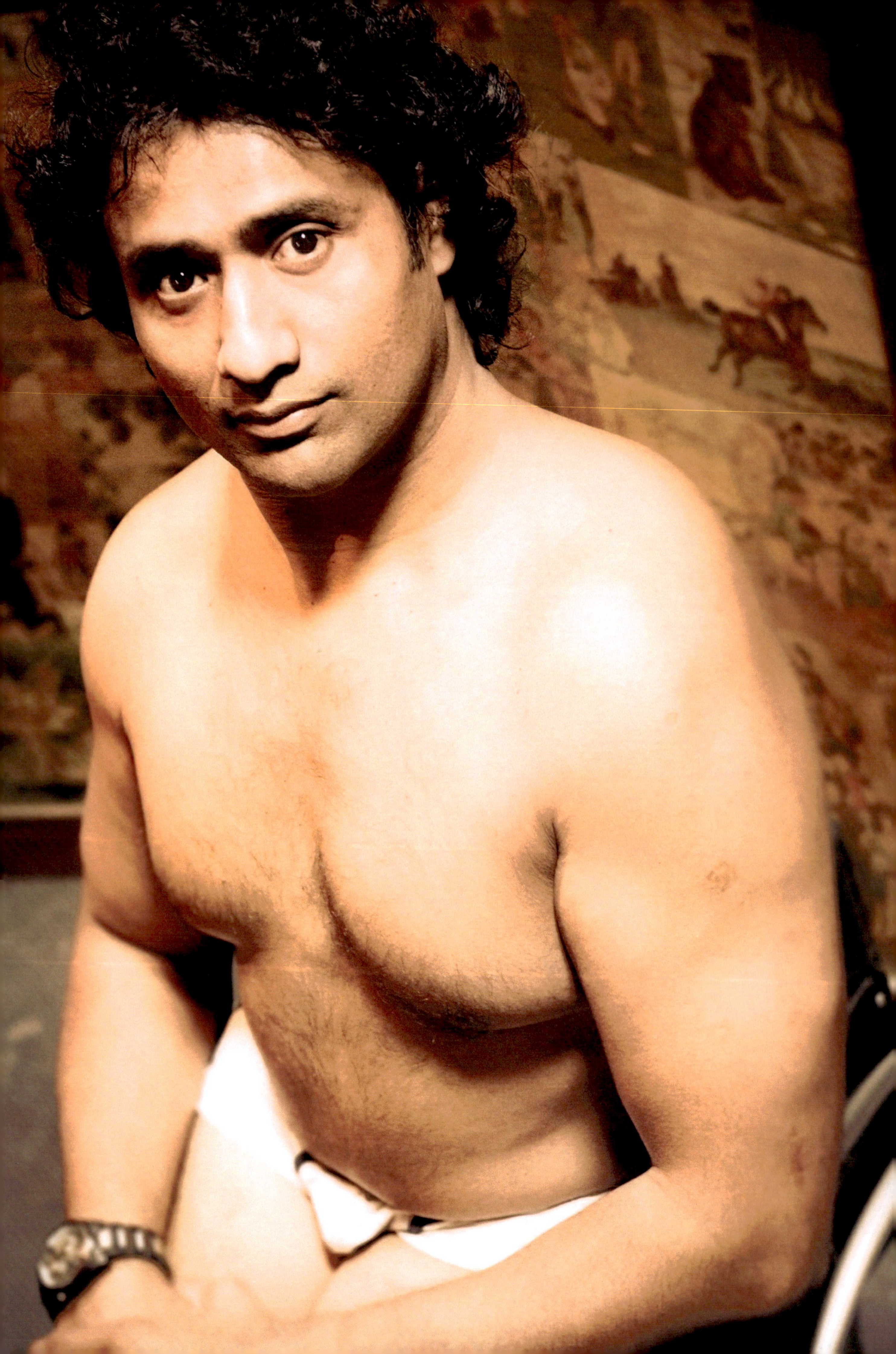

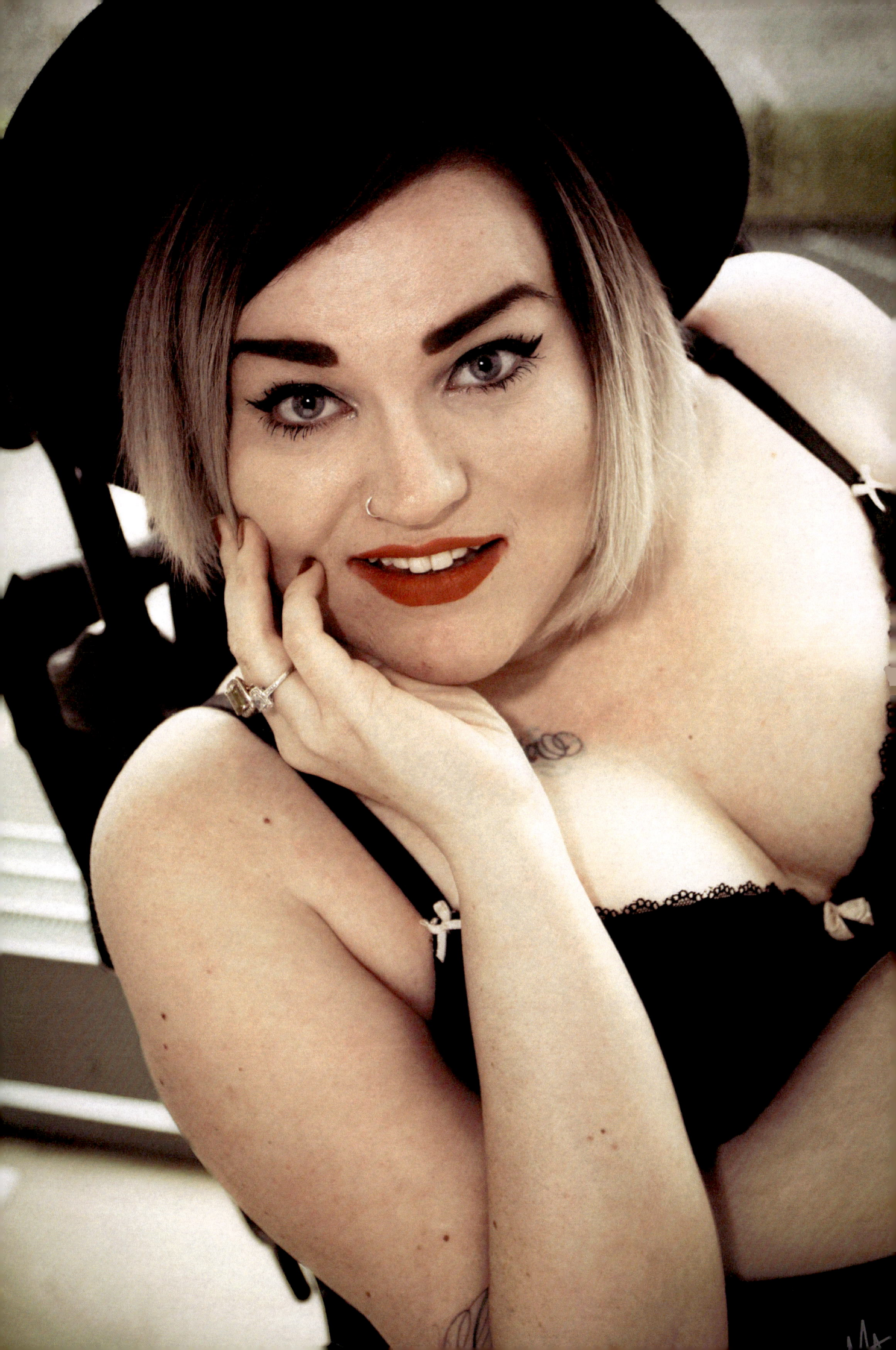

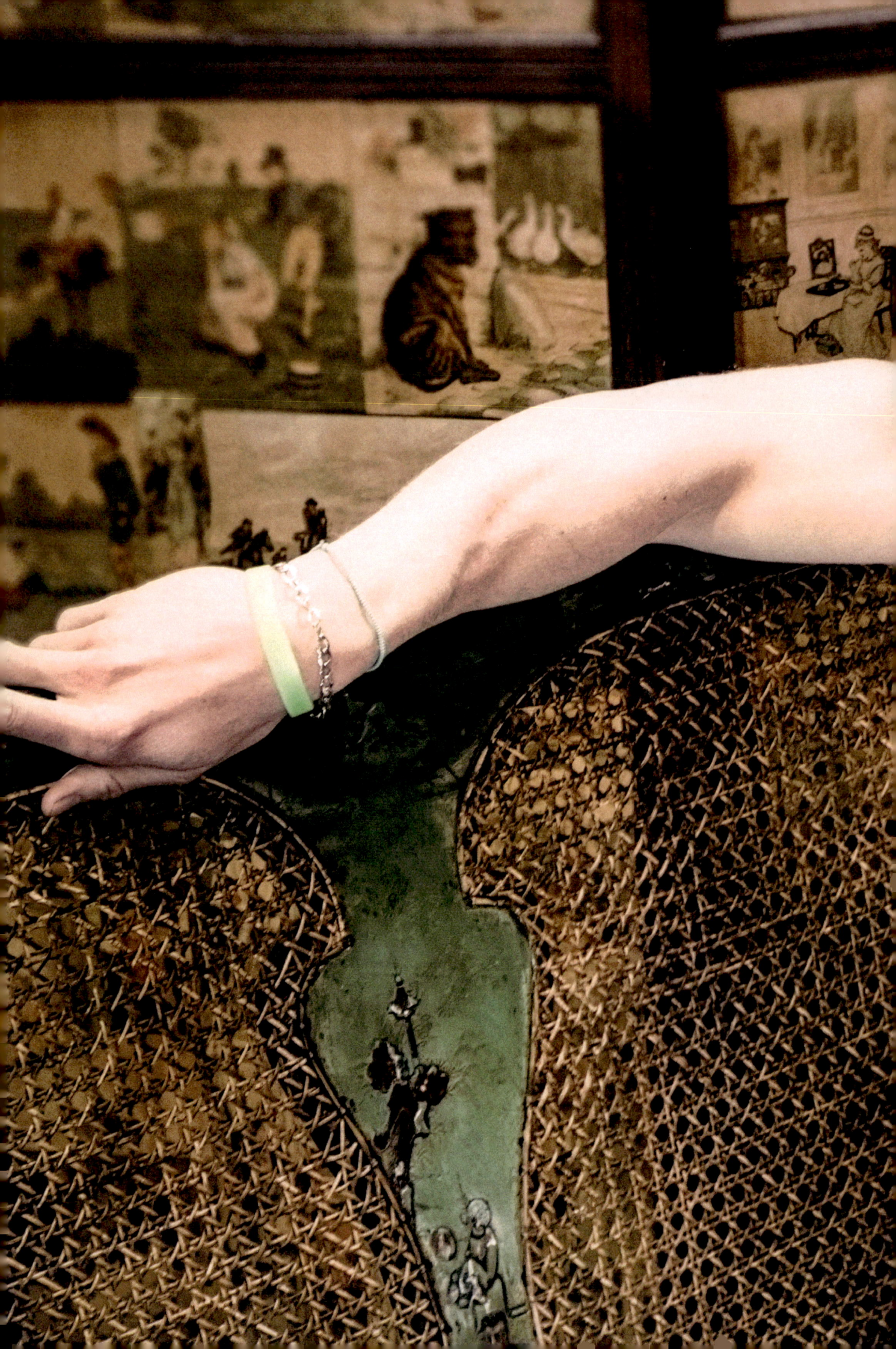

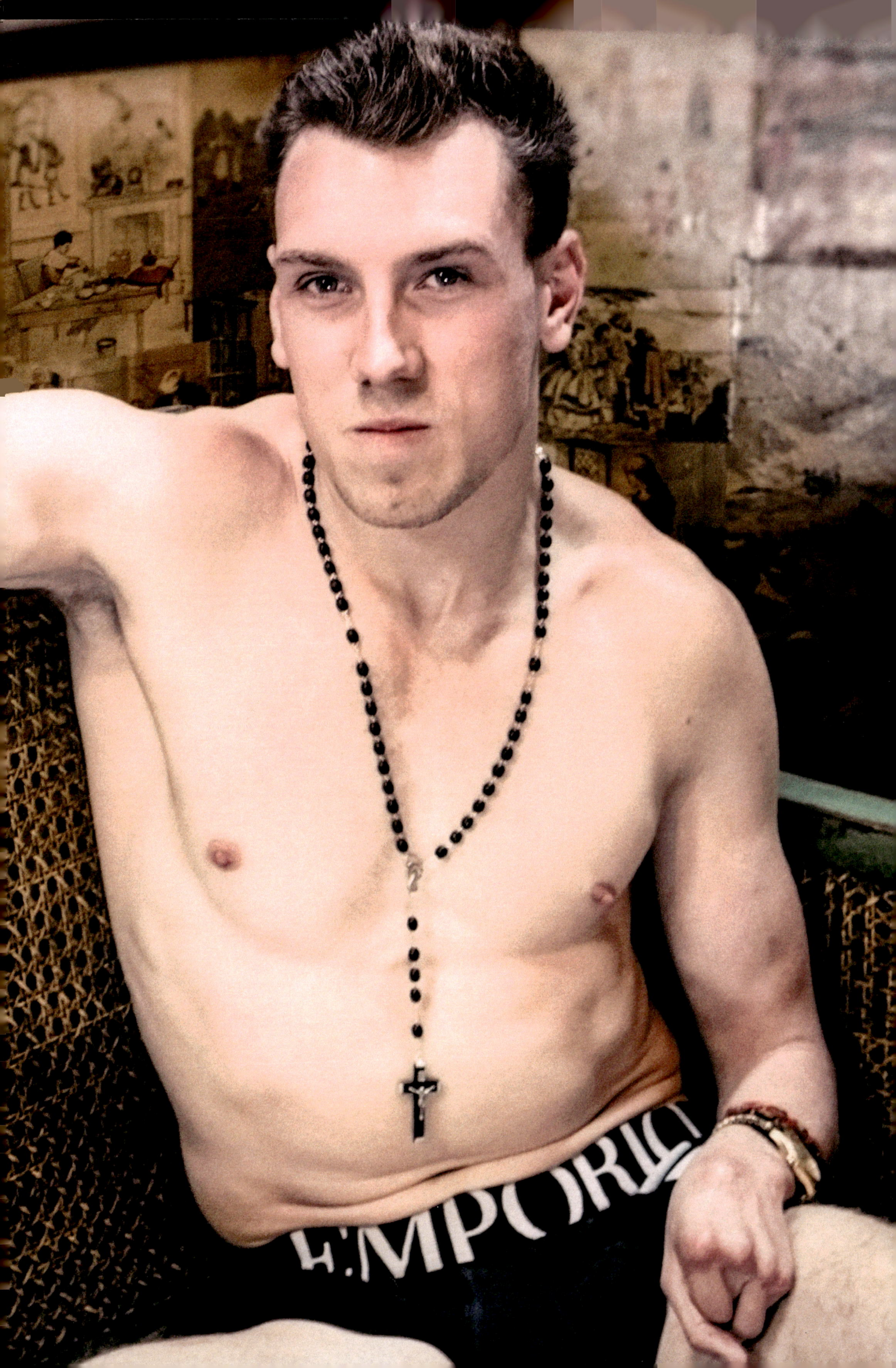

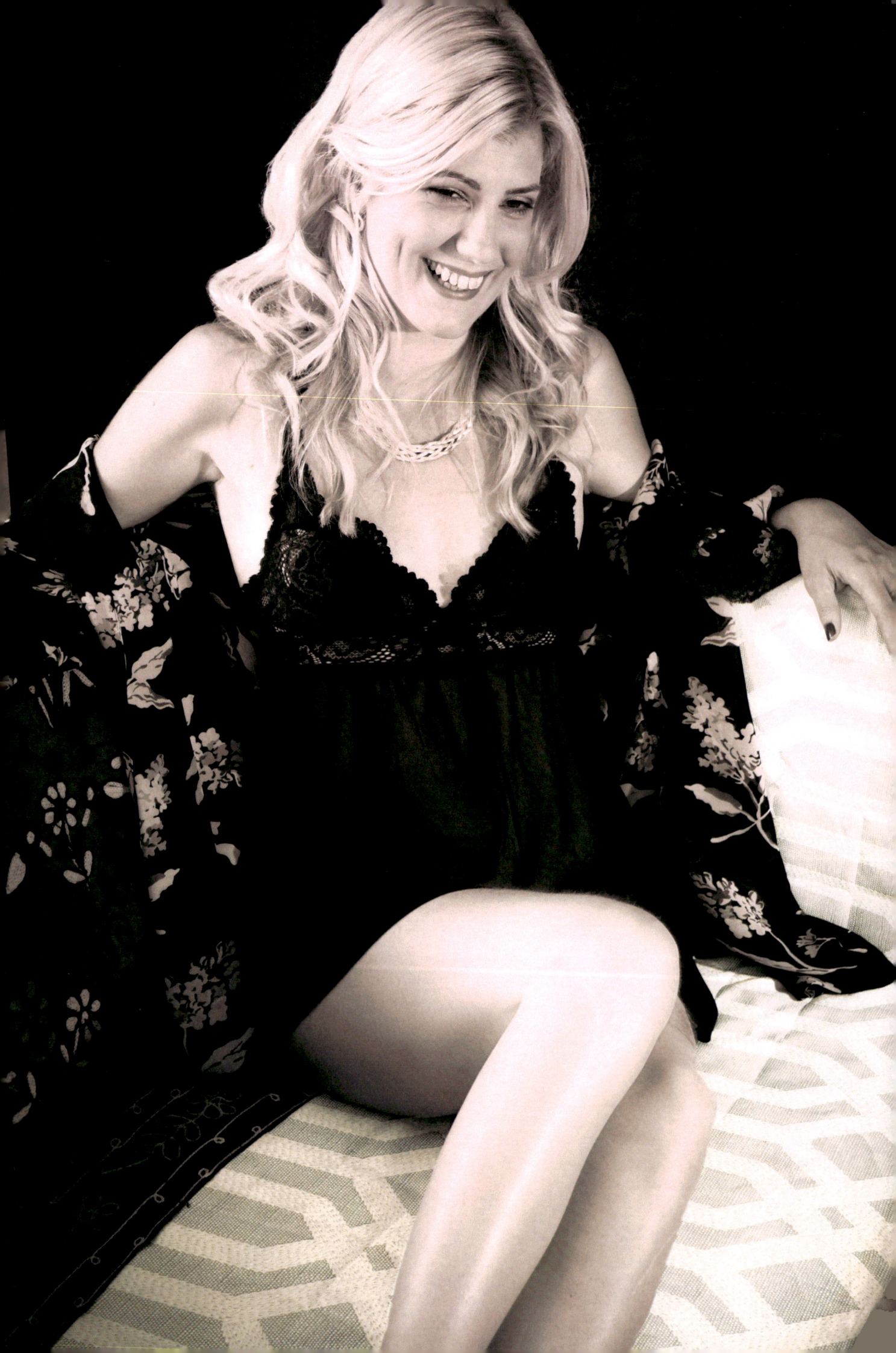

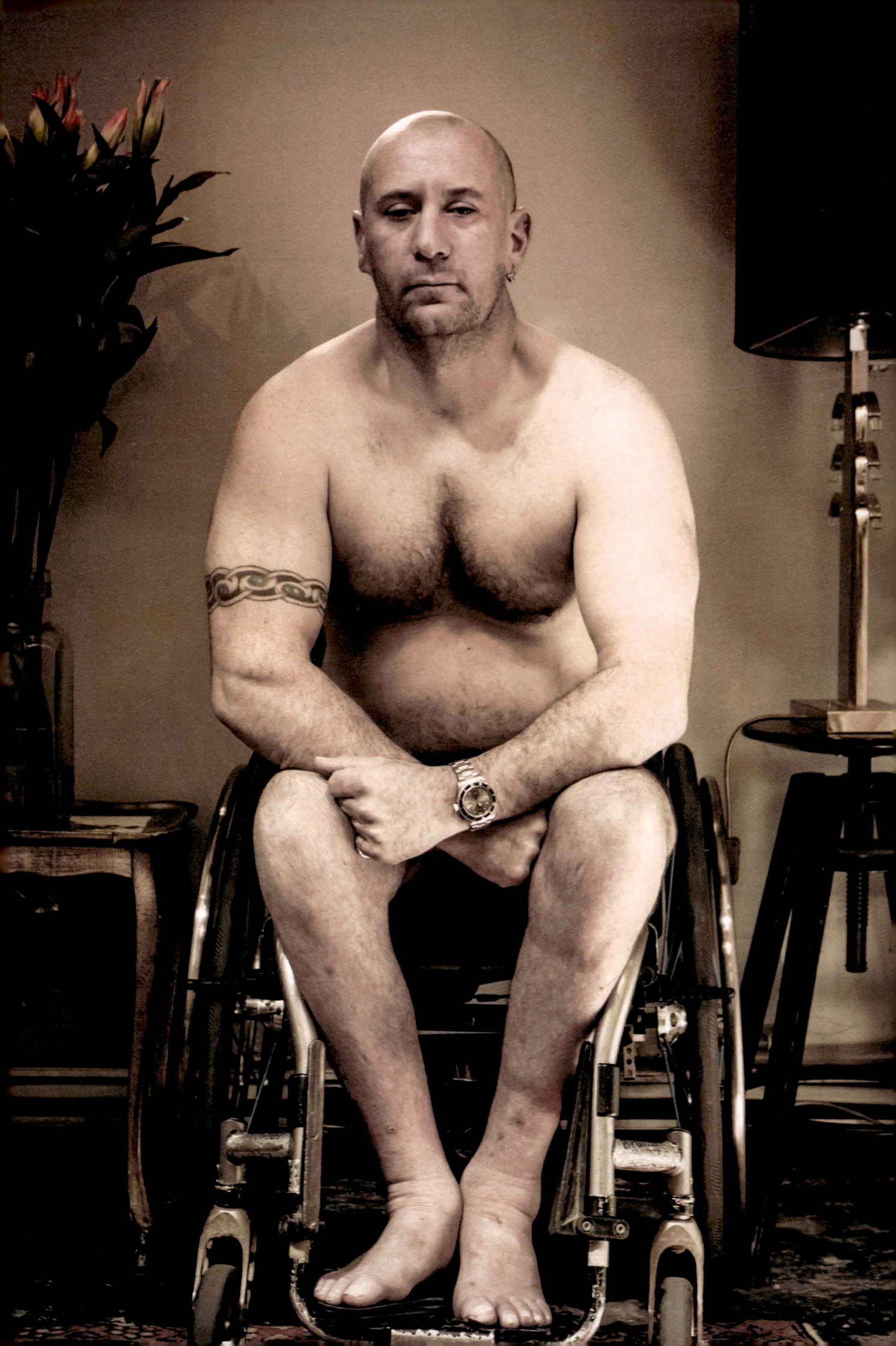

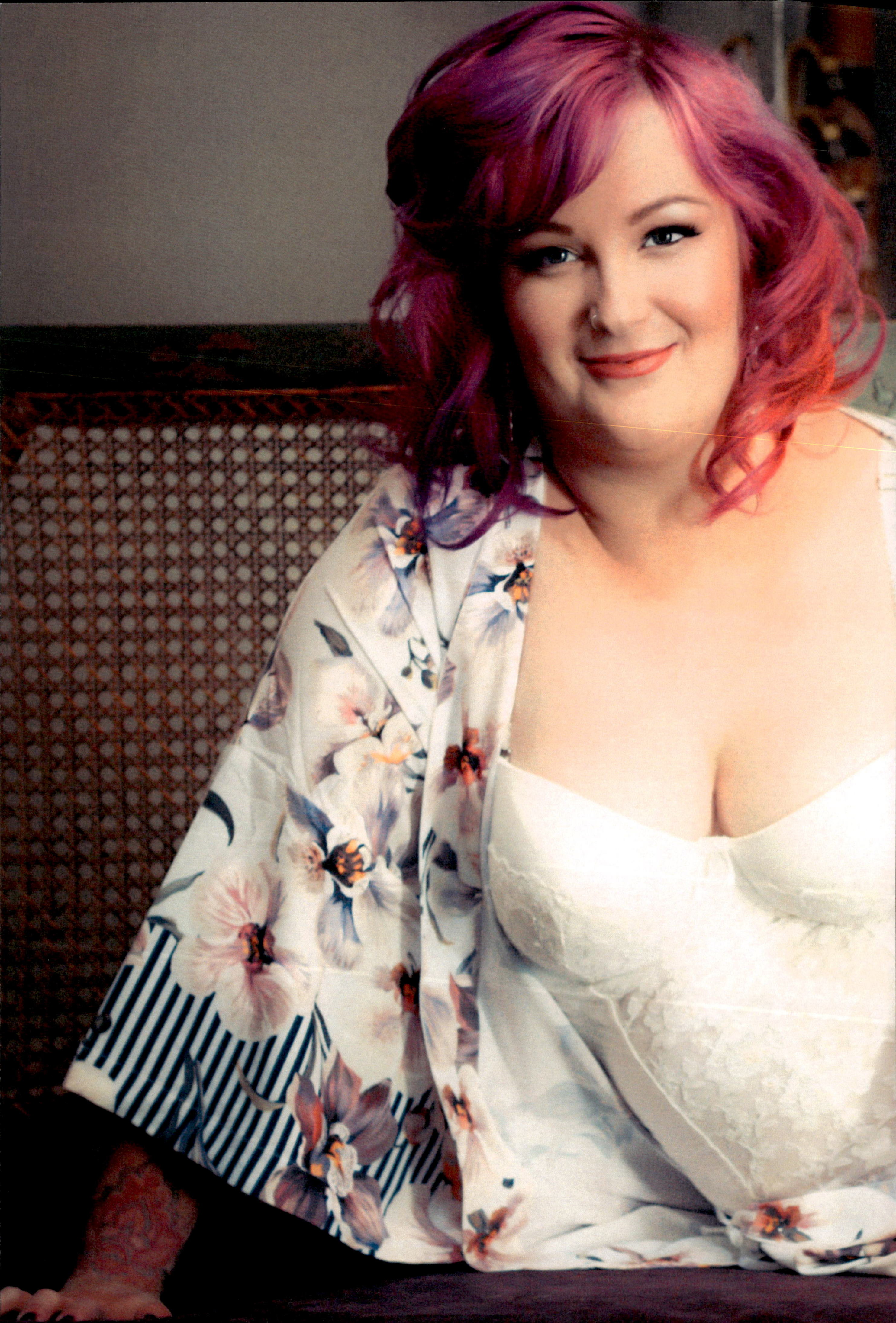

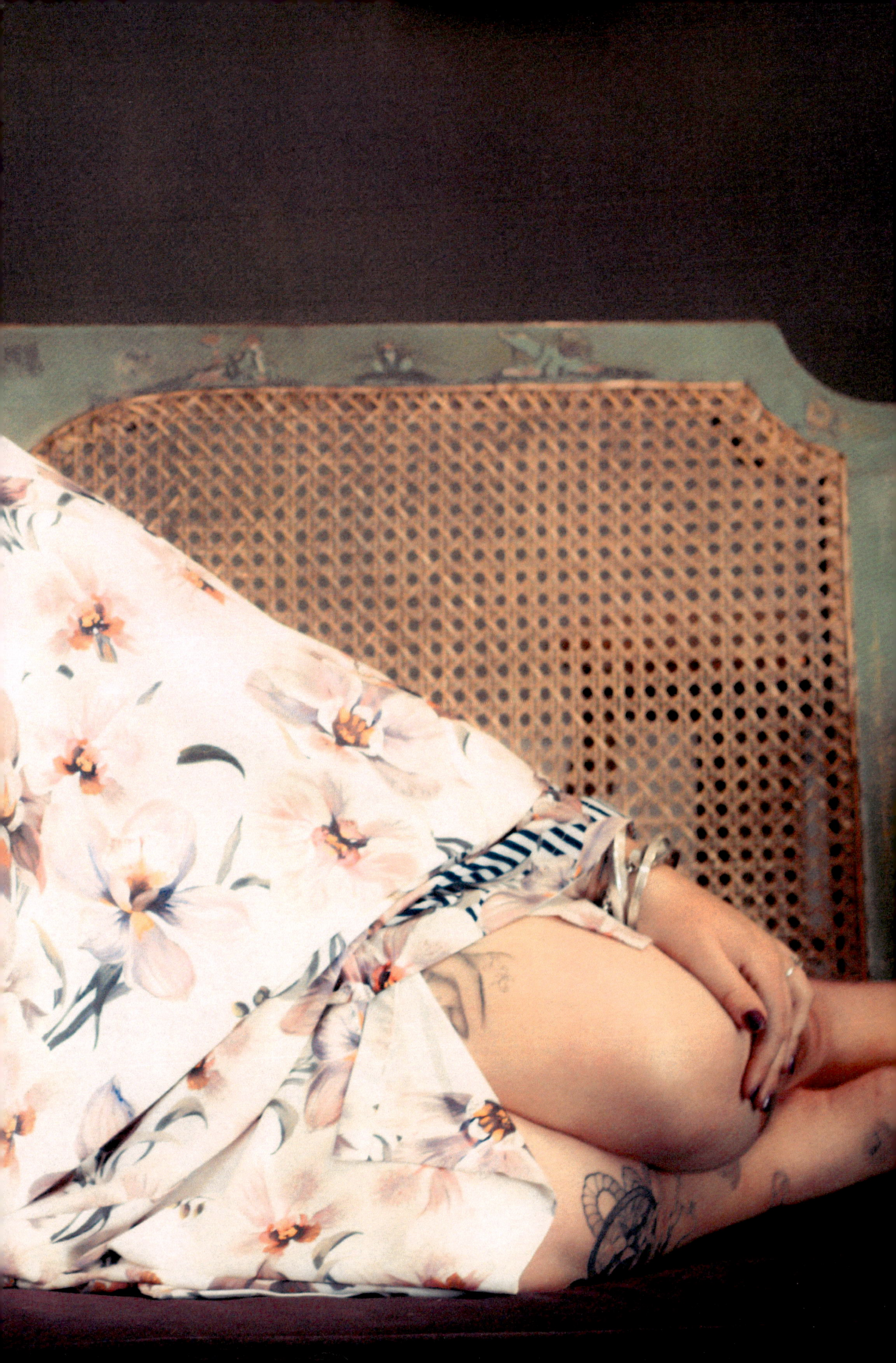

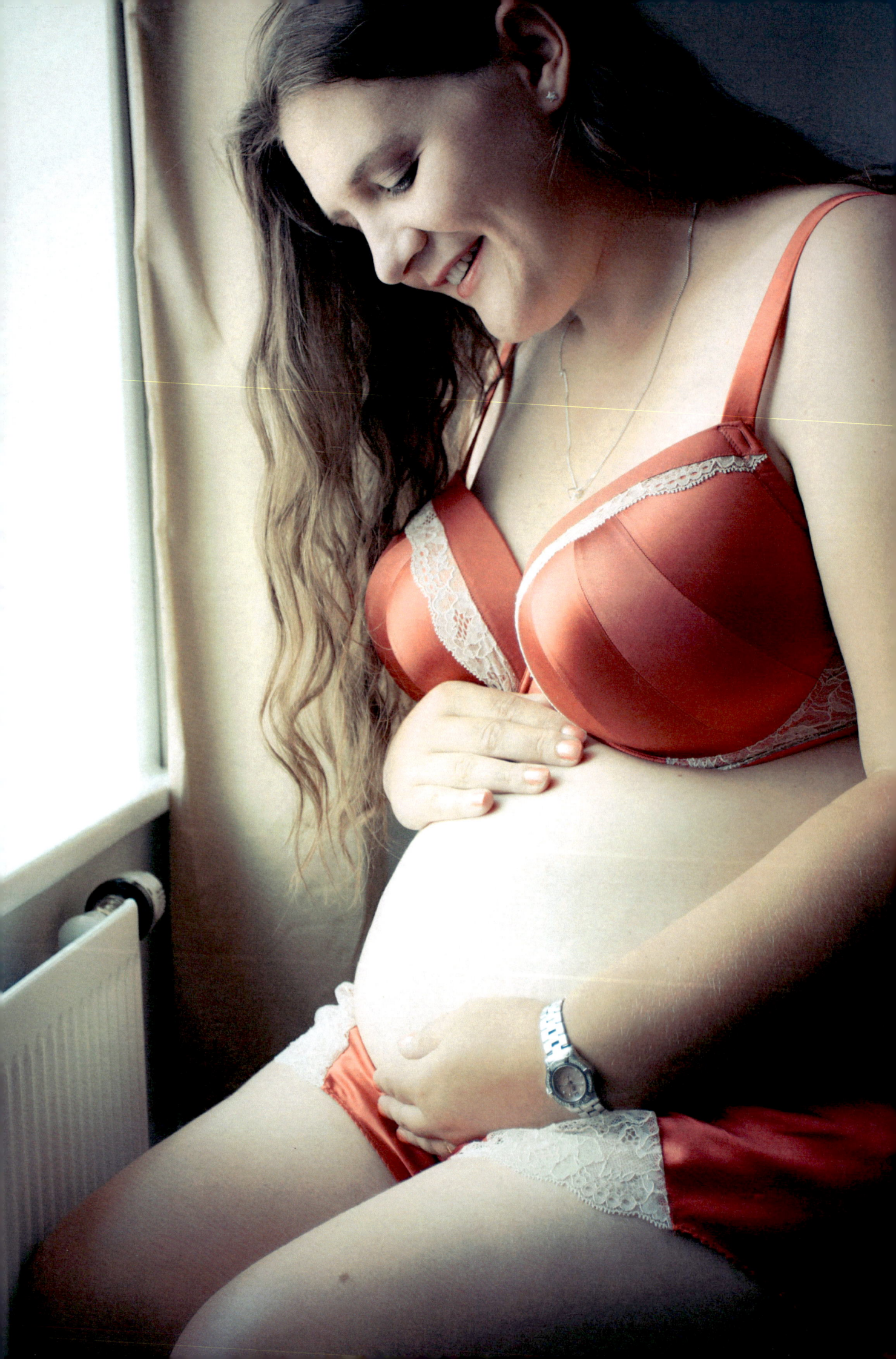

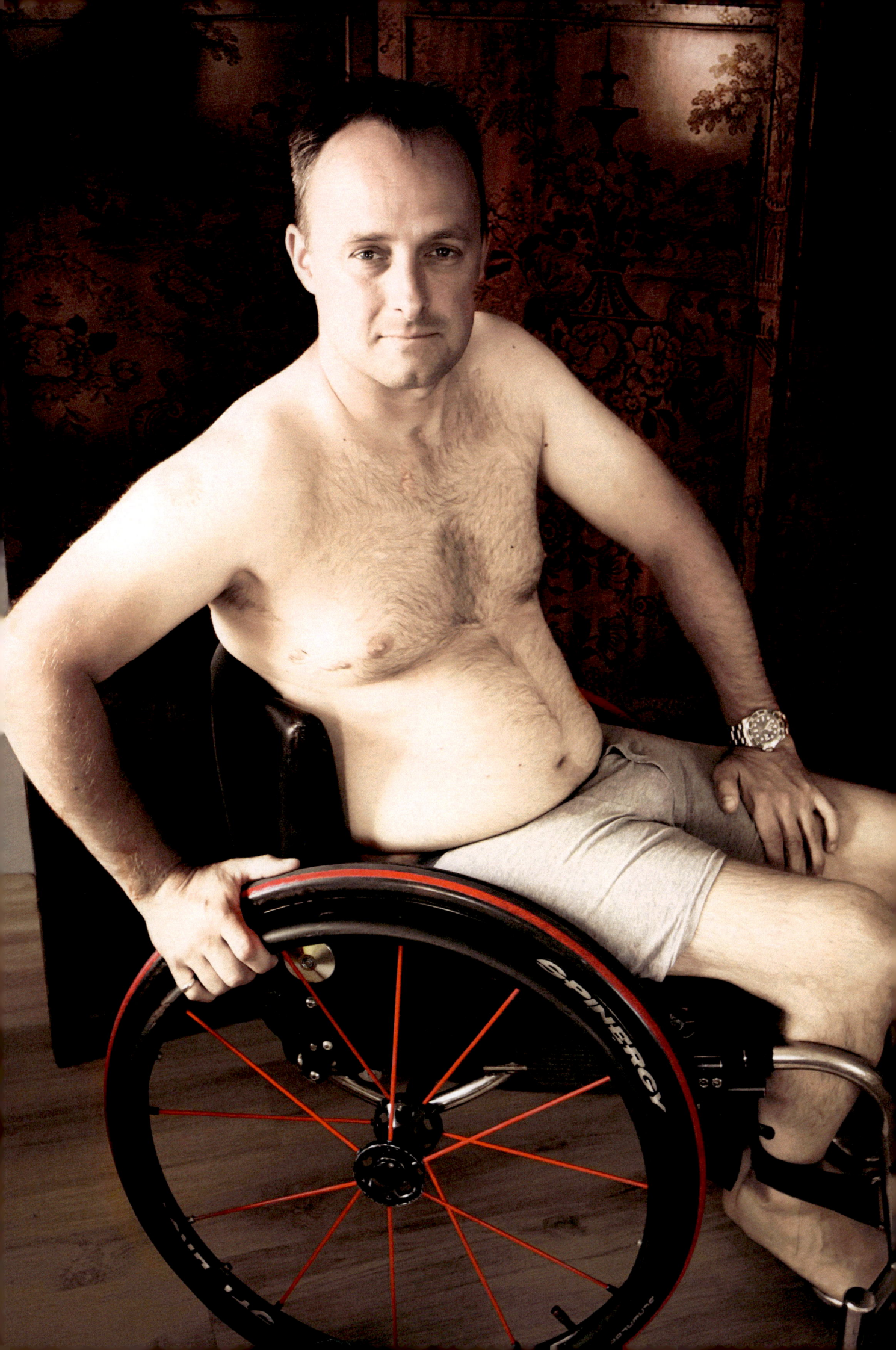

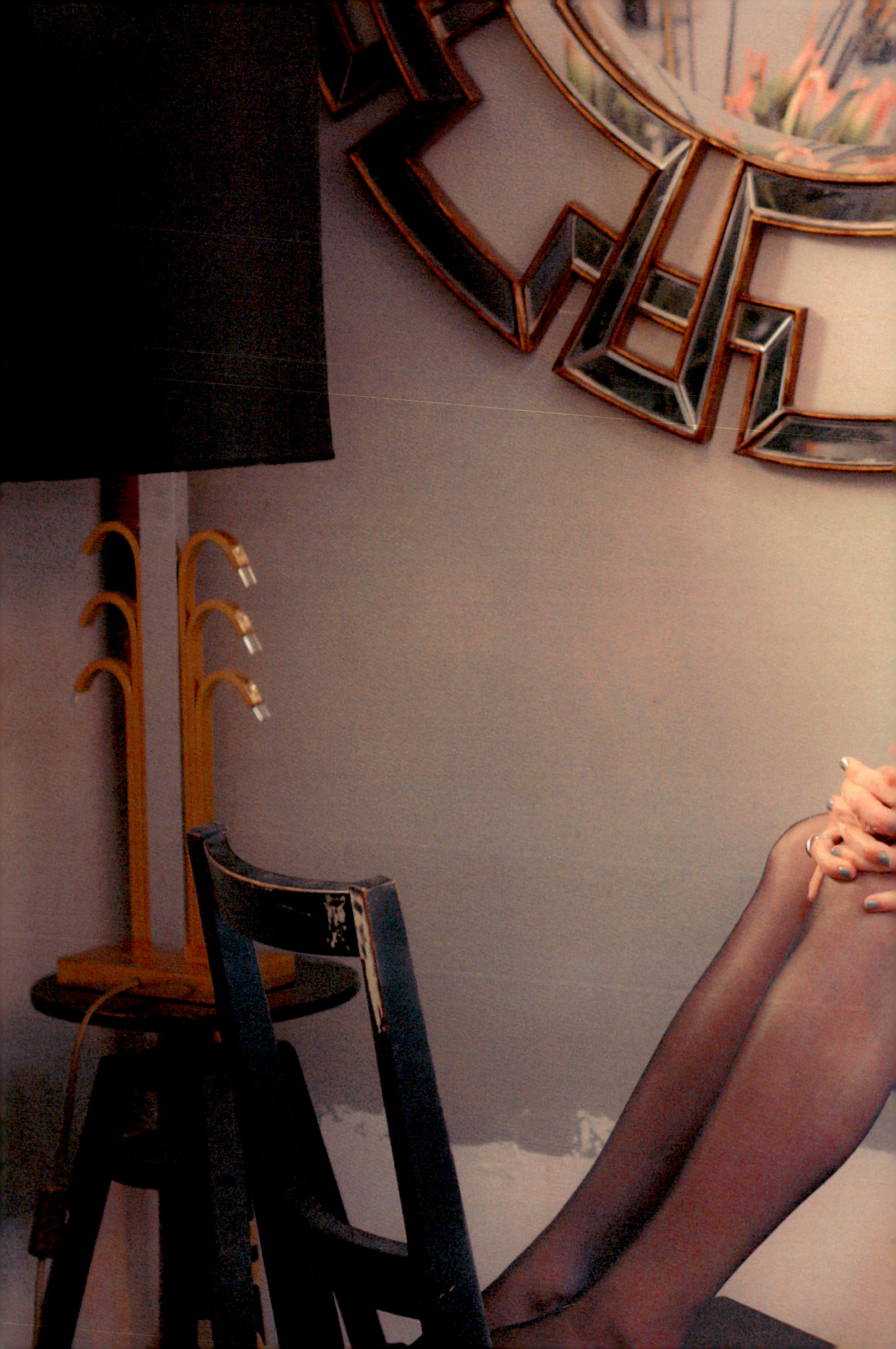

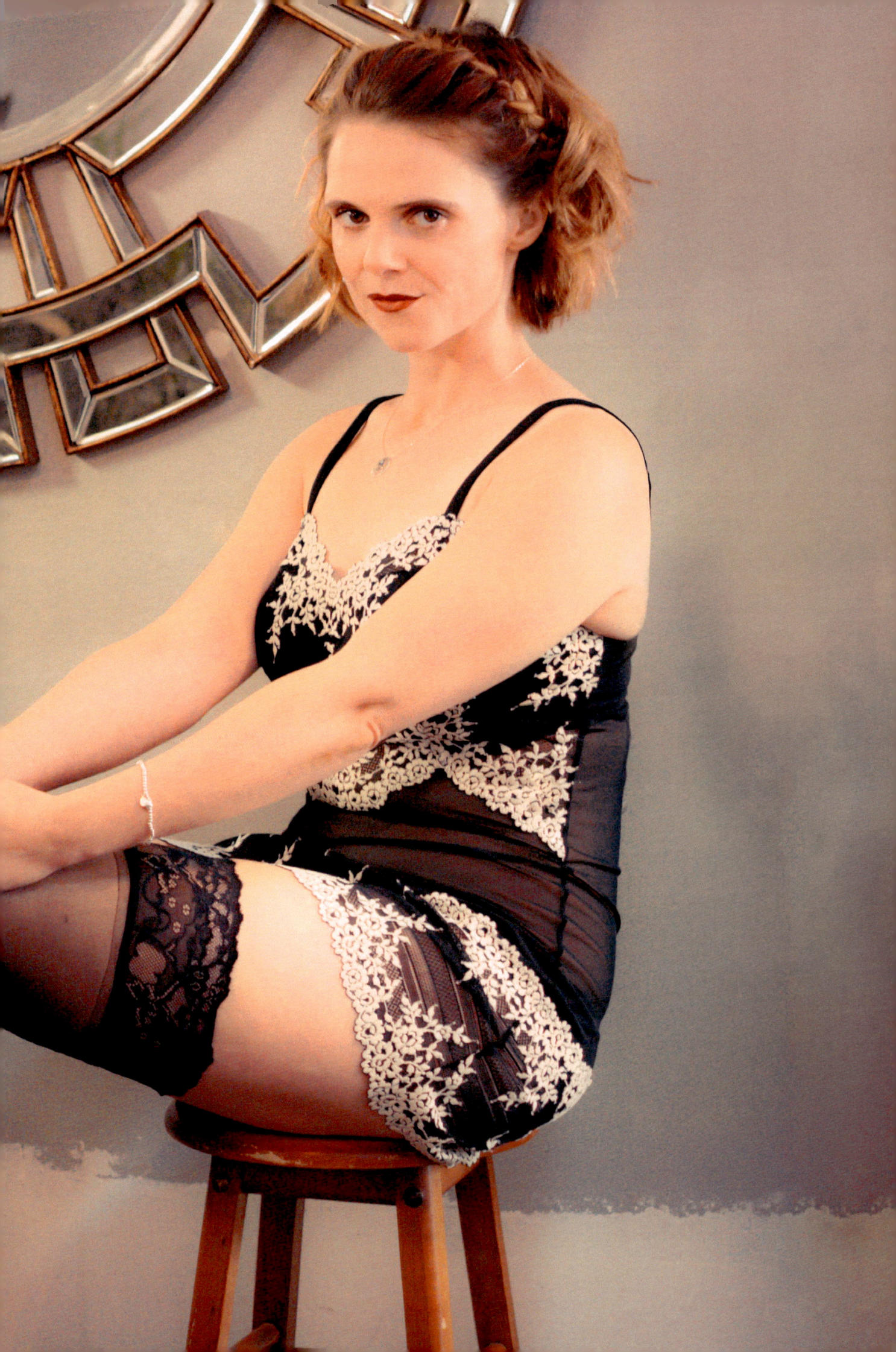

Mary's story

How to describe myself? I'm 46 years young, a bit of a serial dater, empathetic to difference, and promoter of all creatures great and small. To anyone that asks, I just tell them I'm a walking Mary! I was born with a genetic condition called achondroplasia. Fully grown at 4ft 1ins, I never considered myself as different, although society may beg to differ. You might have seen me on 'The Undateables,' and people always comment on how vibrant I am, but I'm just doing me.

I like style, fashion and romance, just like the next person. I think of myself as mildly narcissistic! That's because for far too long I have lived a self-deprecating lifestyle. I was denied the experience of dating, simply because I wasn't considered appealing enough, and I spent much of my time being all too aware that I was the ugly duckling amongst my swan-like friends. 100% effort still didn't even get me to the express checkout with the boys! I reluctantly took my second place title, but secretly knew the crown would be mine one day.

I grew up in Huddersfield but was definitely made in London. I've learnt to take the bitter with the sweet in life, and knew something had to change when my only role models with dwarfism were in the circus. How depressing is that?! Those were my aspirations, and that wasn't who I wanted to be. My warm personality has always helped me and my battle with society. As one of nine siblings, and the only one with dwarfism, it was thought that my personality would only ever be as big as I was. How things have changed!

My dwarfism is the epitome of what I'm about. I embrace it, and will continue to do so. My dipsy nature is what gets me through life, but my Attention Deficit Disorder (ADD) might just be my downfall. In fact, I love everything about myself but that. At times, it appears to be winning the fight, but I intend on winning the war! I feel like I know plenty but just can't retain sweet f*** all! I would never change my dwarfism but I would move mountains to rid myself of ADD – probably something that is a huge surprise to many.

I am a huge person temporarily trapped in a smaller than average sized body. So far, it has served me well...

My employment history is short (pardon the pun), not because I was work shy, quite the opposite! I grew tired of potential employers remarking on my height. Constant questioning, sentences starting with How? Why? Tell us..... To hell with that! The only answer I was looking for was 'you're hired!' Nothing within my height stopped me from doing the tasks that were required. One of my earliest memories was my interview at Pound Stretcher. The list of reasons why they couldn't take a chance on me was as long as the M25 – but all they really needed to say was 'you are just too short to join our team, lady'! I walked out of that interview with my well-protected exterior in tatters... It was the start of a snowball of job rejections. My reply to them was, 'you chose to stunt my growth when you denied me access to the workforce.' I grew tired and looked at other options.

College was a place I enjoyed and felt suitably placed. You only need a brain and determination to join this club. I definitely had determination, but a brain that concentrates and can hold a reasonable attention span was hard for me to acquire! It's definitely healthy, but it sometimes malfunctions. My endless attempts at college should in itself get me a gold medal. I've spent years questioning what is wrong with me; from the outside you see something quite profound and obvious: 'dwarfism.' For me, I see a ball of confusion, anxiety and failure to thrive. For many years my dwarfism has been a small distraction to the bigger problem, and I have been able to hide well beneath it.

When I first moved to London at the age of 21, my condition became invisible. I'd always been the 'wingman' for my friends, protecting them when they got stood up and never expecting that I'd be playing the dating game. But all of a sudden, there they were! Guys telling me they thought I was hot instead of the usual, 'Oh, if only you were a few feet taller' line that I always got in Yorkshire. I felt sexy and would happily return the favour, telling men I met that I thought they were 'a bit of alright'. How can a place only 175 miles south from my home town exhibit and embrace difference so well?

Riding high on a wave of euphoria, I lost sight of my priorities. Ideally I should have solely concentrated on my education; instead I tried to juggle the two, and allowed romance to darken my experience. I met my first boyfriend and had a shotgun wedding. I NEEDED to show the world that someone wanted to marry me for who I was. I had my beautiful son, who was totally worth any wrong decisions I made in the past as I absolutely adore him, but everything else wasn't. I take my time now when it comes to love; I'm probably exhausted after years of playing catch-up and thinking sex was the most important thing in attraction.

I finally don't need to prove anything to anyone, and that makes me so happy. I am as happy single as I am in a relationship. Yes a healthy relationship is wonderful, but I don't feel like the world is coming to an end if I am not in one.

Of course, neither my dwarfism nor my ADD has prevented me from experiencing some very awkward, very tragic and very lovely moments, especially when it comes to dating.

1. I was sitting with a group of friends at a table which had a long satin tablecloth

draped over it, obscuring my legs. A friend of a friend later joined us, and was completely unaware of my dwarfism (and I don't make a habit of announcing my condition). As I stood up to use the restroom, her face said it all: a totally jaw-dropping moment, and one I still remember today! The roar of laughter remains vivid, and always will.

2. One particular dating experience was with a chap who was much more unattractive than his profile picture showed. I am no oil painting, but he knew about my condition as I posted a full length picture of myself. He was less open about his appearance and all was not as it seemed. He politely hinted that, as I was small in height, I'd have difficulty getting a date and therefore he wouldn't mind taking on the challenge. Or so he thought! He picked the wrong girl to mess with…

3. In my teens, I had a favourite nightclub that I'd visit every week just to see the beautiful face of one of the fittest guys in town. He was full of fun and always courteous. One night he said to me 'fuck Mary, you are fit! If only you were taller…' Whilst that was the biggest compliment a guy had paid me to date, it was also the biggest kick in the teeth I'd ever received. I was like a kid with candy that had suddenly lost it all. I am happy to report that these days it takes much more than a 'one liner' to convince me of your affection. The joys of being a naive 18 year old!

4. My first online dating experience was an eye opener. A 'faux pas' I do not wish to repeat anytime soon. I stupidly opened an account and posted information about myself, failing to include a profile picture or mention that I have dwarfism. A certain guy quickly showed interest. His profile picture wasn't earth-moving, but his personality shone through, and we started exchanging emails. Things were going seemingly well…until he asked to see a picture of me. Shock horror! I obliged and quickly hit to send button before I could back out. Wishing I could physically grab that 'send' making its way through the atmosphere, I sat there nervously and waited for his reply. Would he find me shocking, odd, confusing and different? I waited seven whole days for a reply. His response rate prior to sending the picture was almost immediate. Say no more. He basically blamed his hectic work schedule for the delay (excuse number one) then proceeded to add that this dating malarkey may not really be for him after all – but he felt the need to redeem himself and show some sort of empathy towards me, so offered to hook up at some point, for a chat. The hook up never happened, of course. So that was the end of that. The vulnerability and upset that I felt remains palpable. Lesson learned: I always show a full length picture and explain my condition from the start now. Love me, love my dwarfism!

5. On nights out with friends, there is always one, isn't there? In a bar, a drunk guy turned to me and said 'Core blimey! You are the heavens' answer to my perfect 'blow job!' Charming… Well, at least I know if nothing else goes to plan, there is a job for me out there after all!

I've always had quite a distorted view about sex, but that didn't stop me nominating myself as the local agony aunt when I was younger, especially after a few 'girly chats' that got me interested. My qualifications? Truth was I knew diddly squat! I was just a good listener and threw caution to the wind with the occasional sexual innuendo. Like every other woman, I wanted my sexual experiences to be explosive, but interestingly my fantasies never included a 'dwarf' man – how my anxiety might've lessened if they had! Instead, it was always the tallest man with a big package that I thought about. I've always liked a challenge…One thing that I've learnt to love about myself is the 'girl next door' image that my dwarfism seems to give me. It's exciting to be seen as innocent, even more so when I know that's not what men have thought of me when we've been behind closed doors. Nothing wrong with a bit of juxtaposition in the bedroom! I'm also the perfect woman to play out the 'office sex scene', and have done several times with my boyfriend. Being 4'1 definitely has its advantages – one of them being that lovely lift onto the desk just as the fun starts. And of course the positions are only a part of the whole sexual experience. Missionary is great for eye contact, but not so good for me when it comes to comfort – body weight becomes a big issue when you're only my size! I do love receiving oral sex as little positioning or movement is required; I can just lay back and enjoy the ride!

Admiring glances wherever I go is one thing, but a secure relationship is quite another. Only when I am in the comfort of my blanket will I truly let go of my sexual inhabitations.

I'm now at this stage in my life where I'm comfortable enough to freely explore and try things outside the box. Once upon a time I always thought the square pegs only fit in the square holes. Now, round holes with squares pegs – who gives a damn as long as it makes you happy? I do whatever feels natural and I don't worry if a particular position doesn't work for me, it's all about the pleasure! In return I expect to be made to feel like I am the only girl in the world… but who wouldn't want that?

So, where am I now? Well, it'd be great to tell you that I am happily married with 2.5 children and a house in the country. Not yet! What I do have is new found confidence, spunk and aspiration. 'Dwarfism Beautiful' is a name I christened myself and named my Facebook page. It symbolises that we people with the condition are fighting back against the prejudice levelled against us, especially regarding beauty. For far too long we have been the butt of many jokes and the 'last bastion of acceptable prejudice' – even Peter Dinklage, Hollywood actor, says so. The word dwarfism is not commonly associated with beauty, and in fact is often used to represent quite the opposite. I am determined to change this, by introducing people with dwarfism to modelling and beauty campaigns. Ellie Simmonds and Warwick Davis are doing great things, but they are just two people in this country. There are over 6000 people in the UK with dwarf related conditions. So forgive me if I am not overjoyed by seeing only two of them on our TV screens. Beauty, as we know, is not just the outside: something I am all too aware of. I want to challenge the misconceptions, that people with dwarfism cannot be seen as visually beautiful. Let's be honest, it is a title we have lived with for decades. We already know people with dwarfism are academics, medics, entertainers and actors. Let's see how we far we can go when faced with yet another challenge: modelling!

My passion for life is contagious. These days I realise I am inexplicably lucky to have survived decades of struggle and my own depression. I am blessed to have a wonderful son in my life, Reece, who is caring and undeniably handsome to the core. He is my (sane) right hand man. Together we have developed a huge bond, partly because of my single handed mothering, but also because we believe in each other. We encourage each other's dreams and ambitions. I provide the direction and platform for Reece to grow and develop, and in return he gives me hope, confidence and the ability to believe I can succeed. We are partners in crime, the best of friends but more importantly, mother and son.

I now know there's a guy out there for me. Once upon a time I couldn't even believe that.

The previous 'me' didn't think I was deserving of love, or even a decent person. But now? Hell YES I deserve it!

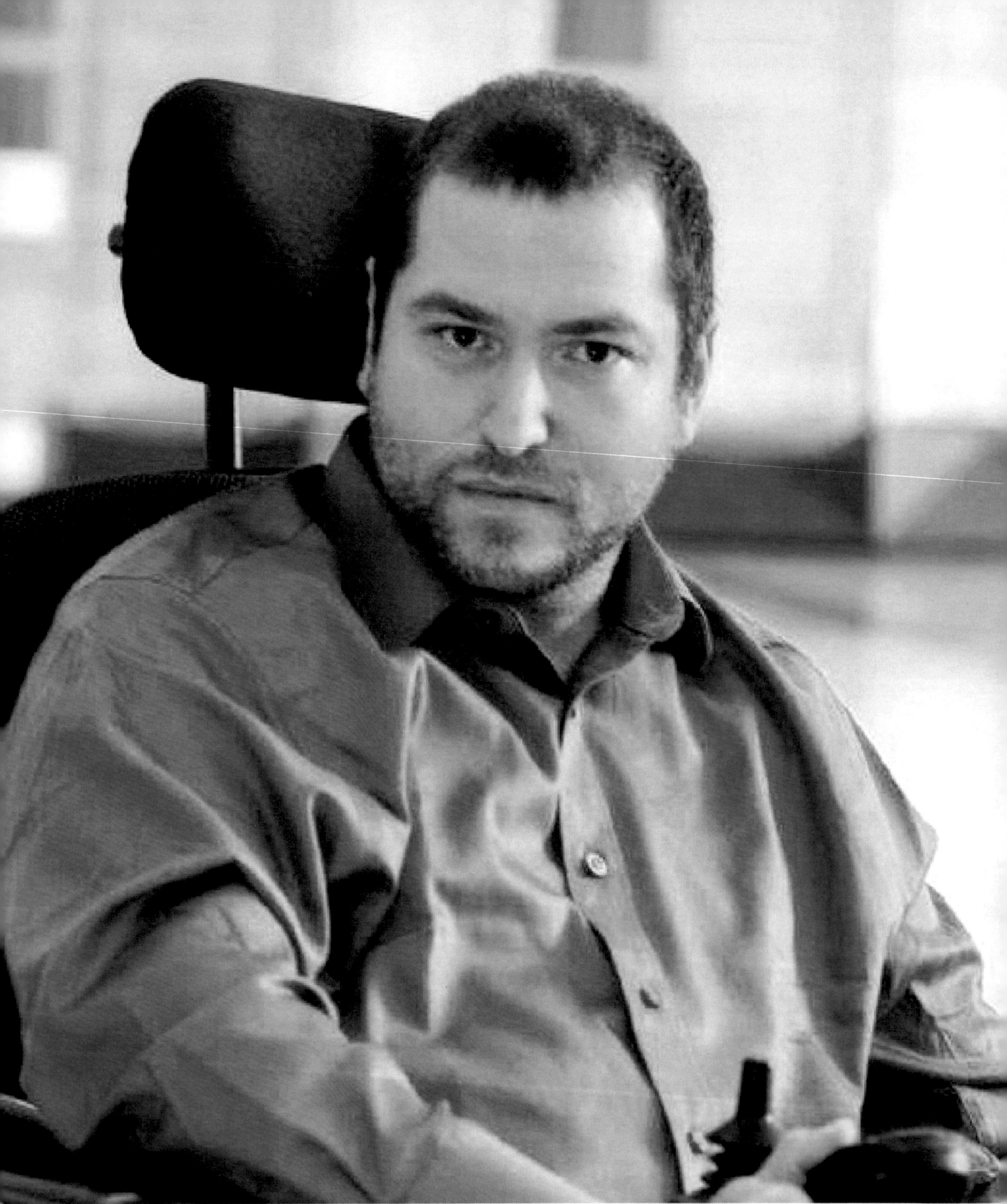

Andrew Morrison-Gurza is a Disability Awareness Consultant with an MA in Legal Studies specialising in Persons with Disabilities. He runs the campaign Deliciously Disabled which aims to create conversations around disability that are based in positivity.

Andrew's story

I remember being 7 or 8 years old and at the local hospital. I was in a heated pool, in an adapted swim class for People with disabilities. I remember that my swim instructor was a young guy, probably around 15 or 16 at the time, with wavy brown hair and a nice smile. During the class, he would hold me in the water and guide me through drills to get me exercising my spastic legs that scissored in on themselves. Every time my swim instructor held me in his arms I would beam at him with a smile that would light up the whole room. I liked being held by him – it made me feel good. That was when I knew there was something different about me.

One afternoon, I decided to tell him how I felt. I proudly announced to him that I loved someone who was in the pool that day. Together, we named everyone in the pool, until the only person we hadn't named was him. "Is it me?" he asked. I exclaimed, "Yup!" and shortly thereafter he was no longer my swim instructor. I can remember feeling that it was something I probably shouldn't have told him.

As I got older and started to understand what being gay meant, I was fairly certain that I was. This realization both excited me and terrified me. I was excited, because it meant that those feelings I had had about good-looking men were valid – they had a name. On the other hand, I was terrified, because I couldn't fathom being both gay AND disabled. Wasn't my life hard enough? I couldn't make it any harder on myself.

As I entered my high school years, I didn't really entertain the idea of dating anyone. I was one of the only students with a visible disability in my school, and I felt that having to deal with that reality was more than enough. So, for the first few years, I said and did nothing in terms of romance, even though, as I rolled through the halls, the feelings and desires grew stronger.

The spring I turned 16, things changed. I had convinced myself that to be normal like my peers I had to start dating. I had been watching a ton of Queer teen romance films in preparation for this. I would watch them over and over again and concluded that, based on the films, if I came out now, the closeted school sports jock would fall madly in love with me and I would assimilate into the queer lifestyle, no problem at all. Le sigh.

I was also reading all the literature around coming out. It kept reminding me that it was "OK to be Gay" and that I was both here and queer. I kept having this gnawing question in the back of my mind, "Was it okay to be Queer AND Disabled?" There was nothing in the pamphlets, websites or movies that gave me the answer. I wasn't so sure, and I remember staying up many nights before coming out, worried that this was all too much to handle.

When the day finally came, and I addressed my sexuality with my family, they were all very accepting of it. I remember my mom renting Priscilla Queen of the Desert that night, and knowing that this part of my identity was OK. For the next couple of years, I grew into my Queer identity with pride. I still hadn't a clue how my disabled identity would factor into all this, but I would soon find out.

Up until university, my identity as a gay man was nothing more than a label that I used to describe my sexual preference. I would use the term gay, but I had no real frame of reference for the experience. Growing up in a small town, and needing help with just about everything as a result of disability, meant that I had no access to the people and places that would help me shape this identity.

When I finally moved away from home, I was determined to find out what being Queer was really all about. One night, I went to a gay club in town. I was so excited – this was my chance to really be gay, and I was going to revel in it. I got dressed up to look as masculine as possible; jeans that accentuated my bulge (they looked great, but sitting in a chair and wearing jeans hurt my manhood more than you will know), a tank top that showed off my muscles, and a hat, perfectly cocked to the left. I wanted to emulate the hyper-masculinity I had seen in gay media and, subconsciously, to draw attention away from my disability so that I could get laid.

As I neared the club that night, I envisioned my entrance: throngs of gay men around me as I rolled in, in my wheelchair, just waiting to dance with me. When I got there, however, I learned I had to enter the club through the back and use the service elevator to get on the dance floor, effectively killing that fantasy. I remember being overwhelmed by all the good-looking men that were also gay. I was excited to talk with all of them.

As I wheeled closer, taking a deep breath and diving into the fray of well-sculpted bodies before me, I noticed that each and every one of them moved back as I moved further in. At that moment, the two identities that I had worked so hard to shape separately, crashed in on themselves. I realized, that in this space I wasn't just gay, I was also disabled. It became clear to me then that disability wasn't a part of the gay experience. After seeing the way they looked at me, unsure of whether to move out of my way or not, I came to understand that I would have to come out in a whole different way than I had before. I would have to come out as disabled.

Growing up, I always knew that my disability played a role in my life; it was undeniable, I was a little kid in a 300-lb. chair. My family did a really good job of incorporating my disability into their lives; they traveled with me everywhere, included me in every activity, and never really made my disability a life-altering thing. In that way, I never really thought much of it, it was just second nature – until now.
All of a sudden, my queerness was not the issue. My identity as a Person with a

Disability was. Every time I liked a guy, wanted to go on a date, or get laid, I would have to come out of the closet and down a ramp, crashing smack dab into my crippled identity. I would constantly worry that they would see just how disabled I was, and reject me because of it. My fears were not unfounded, and my disability often denied me the connections I craved. I did everything I could to force the two identities apart, failing to realize the more I did so, the more they became intertwined.

One such instance, highlighting this inextricable bond between Queer & Crippled, came one night during a hook up. I had just spent the evening with an adorable exchange student. Everything had gone swimmingly; he was cute, considerate and not afraid of the wheelchair and all that entailed. We had just finished, and he went out in the bathroom to pee, closing the door behind him. Normally, this would not have been a problem, except that he had locked the door behind him, leaving me flat on my back in bed unable to move and assist him in any way. As I lay there while he fiddled with cutlery trying to get back in, I realized just how linked these two identities were. If I weren't disabled, I could open the door for him, but here I was in the "dead turtle position", locked in my own room with a naked man in my kitchen. The security guard of my building eventually busted through the door, letting him back in, and seeing me in all my glory. We had a good laugh about it, but it is one of those moments that reminds me that my disability will always be there – even when I wish it weren't.

Throughout my twenties, there were indeed failed attempts at intimacy, wherein I perceived my disability to be the problem. I continued to believe that no one wanted to be with me, because I was disabled. I struggled to come to terms with my reality, not wanting to accept what was staring me in the face.

It wasn't until recently, as I entered my thirties, that I began to truly understand that within my disability was the opportunity to create change. One day I was sitting at home bored, clicking through gay websites, annoyed that representation of my body as a Queer man with Disabilities was nowhere to be seen. I wanted more than anything to see myself, or someone like me in gay themed media, so I could be reassured that this intersection in which I lived really was okay.

I started contacting magazines and media outlets, asking to tell my story, and realizing that in doing so I was creating the representation that I craved. One such opportunity came about, and they asked me how I would like to be described in the piece they were writing. I was ready to tell them that I was a Queer Person with a Disability living with Cerebral Palsy, and spout off my standard answer, which by now I had regurgitated many times before. In that moment though, I stopped and cheekily told the reporter that I was "Deliciously Disabled". Right then, something clicked. My two identities made sense to me now. I didn't have to be Queer and Disabled or Disabled and Queer, trying to shove both identities into another. Instead, I had created a new identity for myself that encompassed the reality of my disability and sexuality, together as one.

I have started using the term "Deliciously Disabled", and finally feel that my journey to accept myself is on the right path. I see now that my disability only enhances my sexuality, and vice versa. Now when I open the closet door and slide down the ramp, I do so proudly knowing that my identity as a Deliciously Disabled man is a flavor of the Queer community that has a taste all of its own.

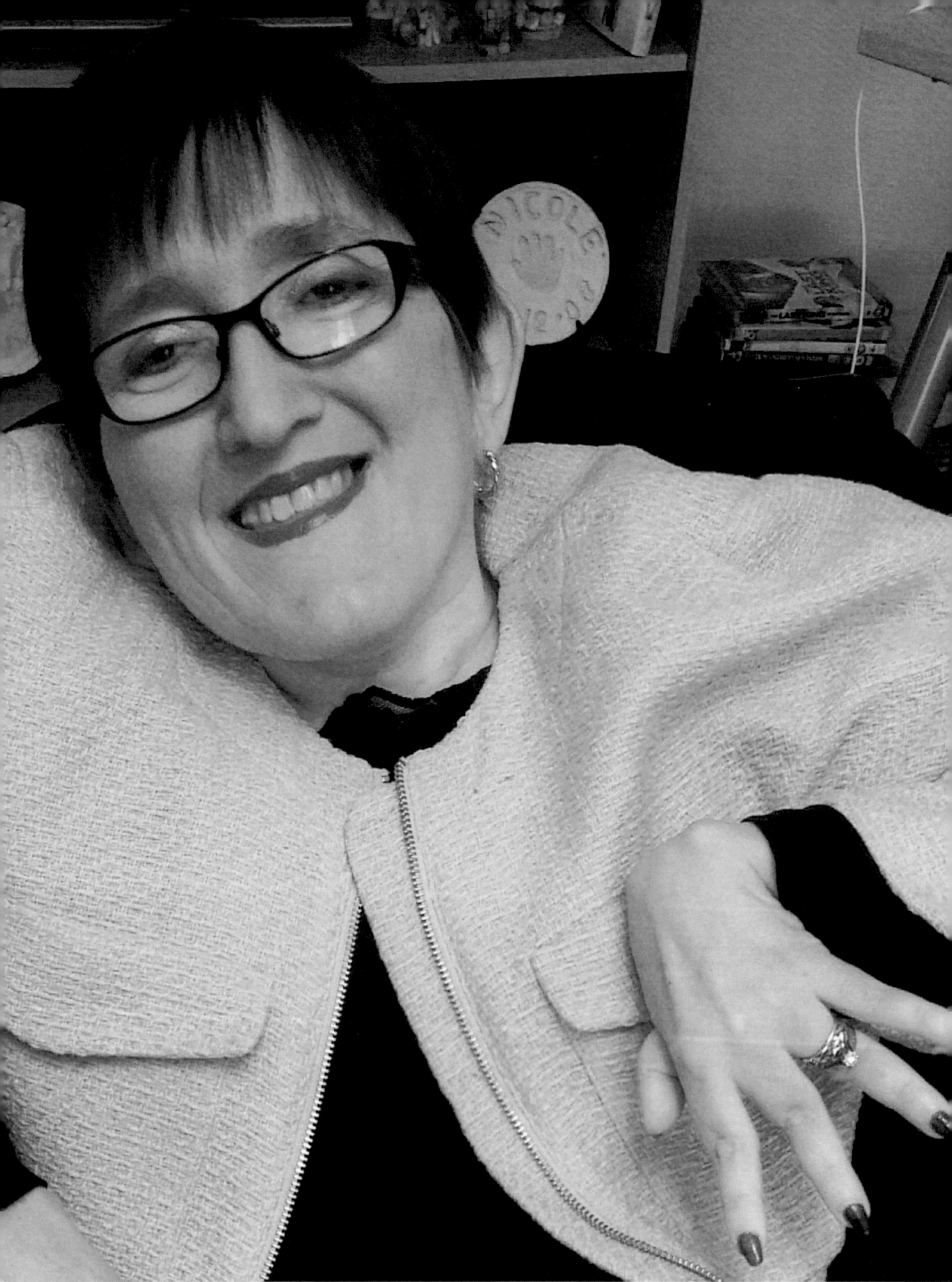

Lynn Kelly is 45 years old and lives in Sunderland, campaigning for supported living. She has severe cerebral palsy and is a quadriplegic.

Lynn's story

The story I am about to tell you is a complex one but one that I hope you will find intriguing, and perhaps will resonate and help anyone finding themselves in a similar position.

My name is Mrs. Lynn Marie Kelly, I'm 45 and I live up North, in Sunderland. I have severe cerebral palsy and am a quadriplegic. I use an electric wheelchair to get around, and live in assisted living accommodation. That basically means that I am supported by care staff, but am practically in my own home and can come and go as I please.

Firstly, I am a widow. It has recently been the ten year anniversary of my husband's death. He was quite a bit older than myself, so I knew to some degree that the time was ticking for the pair of us, but of course that did not prepare me for his loss.

I married Paul in July 1993 and we did have a very strong marriage. He had muscular dystrophy so we were both cared for in nursing homes throughout our relationship. One of our greatest achievements, as a couple, was starting a campaign for supported living in our local area, as it's incredibly important to me that disabled people are able to partake in the local community.

Paul and I did have an intimate sex life of sorts but because of our disabilities, and issues with movement, this was considerably reduced. Basically, our marriage was never fully consummated and I am still technically a virgin. We decided that we didn't want any hands on support from our care staff regarding our sex lives, as we felt this ruined the true intimacy. Ironically, the care we did need involved very intimate care such as bathing, bowel, continence and menstrual care. It may seem paradoxical that we were fine with functions care and not sexual care, but this is how we felt.

However, that would be on the basis that we were offered any sexual care. The truth is that we were not. Even though neither of us wanted it, personally, it would have been nice to have the option, and I'm sure it would be useful to many other disabled couples. Sexuality with disabled people is so often poo-pooed and ignored in society, and that is something I'd like to see changed.

Paul and I dealt with the issue the best way that we could, for example: he would be turned towards me to kiss me goodnight by our care staff. We started out as very good friends and had similar aims in life so that made for a very good marriage. At one point I did stray a little bit and had sexual interest in other men. Paul and I were certainly not a stuffy couple but intimacy wasn't always spoken about between us, and this could be frustrating for me. He said that I could go and find out what I needed to do and he would wait for me. He didn't want me to go without my sexual expression.

I decided that, actually, no, I didn't want to be intimate with other men to that extent. I loved Paul and felt committed to him. That just shows Paul's strength in character to be able to say that to his wife.

So, my marriage on the whole was good. Temptations were there but we got over them. But the reason I took up the offer with this book is because of a situation that started in June 2013. I am going to keep the identity of this person anonymous, so I am not going to mention his name.

I had just been out in my local shopping centre and booked a wheelchair accessible cab with a local cab firm that I trust and still travel with to this day.

I was waiting by the kerb and a cab pulled in. A man around my age came around and started preparing to load me in. He was asking about my chair and we started having a bit of a laugh together. I was winched into the cab, got in and we set off. I started up a conversation since I'm a pretty chatty person. I noticed that he was foreign and asked him if he was Italian. He said, "No, I'm Polish." I said, "Oh." "I'm sorry I'm not Italian", he replied, and we started having a chat. He told me that he had just returned from Warsaw and mentioned the nice hot weather. I churlishly asked him if he had been over to give money to his wife and kids. He said, "No." I then bravely asked, "are you single?" He replied, "Yes." I then very flirtatiously said, "I'm single too. I'll have to get your number." I asked his name and said, "no doubt I'll see you again." This would be a very strong probability since they are one of the only cab firms in the area with cars for my needs. I then proceeded to wander into my house, giggling like a schoolgirl, when my carer asked me if I was okay.

I didn't deliberately book him when I needed a cab, but after that day he often came to pick me up. We had lots in common and liked the same Eighties music. He said he was a music producer and also used to be a policeman in Warsaw, although I'm a bit skeptical about that one.

Now, if you remember, he declared himself to me to be single. And I didn't think anything else of that, as of course you take people at face value when you first meet them. He continued to pick me up in his cab all through summer and our relationship proceeded to blossom.

Our conversations deepened and turned quite explicit. I just knew something was going to happen between us. I was telling my carers all this and although they were pleased for me, they didn't want me to be vulnerable or naive.

One day one of my carers was taking another client out in his taxi and, without my permission, told him that I had feelings for him and that I tend to latch onto people because of what I've been through. He reassured her and told her that he would never do anything to hurt me. She asked him how he felt. He looked her straight in the face and said, "I do like Lynn, very much."

Now, because of the nature of what I do with the housing commission, I often have to go to meetings far away - like Newcastle - and he asked if he could always take me to these meetings. This meant we had a lot of time to talk and by December 2013 we were having a lot of good fun together. We were having very meaningful conversations and I was really opening up to him about my insecurities and how I hate myself in terms of my sexuality.

He kept telling me that there was nothing wrong with me and that I could be with anybody that I wanted. I said, "How can I even reach up and have a kiss with someone? You could go to a club and pick someone or reject someone. I have to say, do you mind if I give you a kiss? I don't know what I can offer to somebody." He was reassuring and would say things like, "Lynn, it takes time…"

On December 4th 2013 I had a housing association meeting in Durham. As usual, he'd taken me. I had developed a girlish plan to see whether or not he truly liked me. At the end of our trip, I planned to kiss his hand and gauge his reaction, then I would finally know for sure. But during our journey he kept saying that he didn't know whether he will see me over Christmas, and this was irritating me.

As I left, I blew him a few kisses to wish him merry Christmas. I realised I couldn't leave yet, as the lights on my chair were flashing. I turned to tell him that my chair was jammed but, as I turned my face, there is another face there. His face. I squealed and his mouth latched on to mine and we were kissing. I placed my good hand on his face and really got into it. I am genuinely and totally surprised. It's been years since my last intimate kiss, and he initiated it.

When I came into my bungalow, I didn't even turn the lights on straight away. I wanted to savour the moment and I didn't want my carers wondering why I was shaking from head to toe. In the days following that moment, I was telling people that there was something there and I really had feelings for him. I thought I was falling in love him. I thought this was the perfect time and opportunity to ask him to Christmas dinner, but he didn't appear.

During all this time I had been asking for his private phone number but he had never given it to me. I had felt this was very unusual considering the nature of our relationship. I decided to go on the dreaded Facebook and found his profile through his record company, which I knew the name of. When I went on his profile, I saw that he was tagged 'in a relationship.' I started seeing stars and I felt really funny.

I got on the messenger service and I demanded that he come over straight away and explain himself. He was round in a matter of minutes. He opened my front door and said, "hello my baby girl!" I said, "never mind baby girl." I screamed, "SIT DOWN," and the rest was expletives. I said, "have you got something to tell me?" He said, "no." I said, "relationship?" And he went, "ahh," while twiddling his thumbs. I was in an utter state of fury and shock.

"Yes, ahh. Who is it?"
"Ahh. Right. Um."
"It better be good. What is it? Wife?"
"No."
"Children?"
"No."
"You're running out of options. I'm WAITING. I WANT to know."
"Um… Um."

Five minutes passed in silence, and by this time he had gone grey. And he said…
"I'm gay."
"You're not gay."
"I'm sorry."
I was hysterical. I felt so betrayed and angry. He continued.
"And yes, I'm with someone."
"Is it new?"
"No, Lynn. We've been together for eleven years. We came from Poland because we were being persecuted against."

At that point my world completely caved in. I had a physical and mental breakdown and had a seizure. My carers rushed in and he went out crying, taking off at a rate of knots. During that conversation, I asked him if he loved me. That even though he has declared himself as a gay man, I asked if he would love me if he was straight. He said, "I do love you, Lynn. I love you very deeply." I said, "listen, save it for someone who cares," even though of course I cared.

He had fallen to his knees and said, "I beseech you, Lynn. Please don't tell anyone." But of course I told everybody. I vented my anger on Facebook, but I didn't realise he could read my posts. I then tried to pull our relationship back but he refused. At this point, I went to go and have counselling since I was also dealing with a family crisis all alone, and was nearly cracking under the pressure. He was still coming round to pick up others in assisted living, so that was extremely hard.

I still felt like I loved the man and felt a sense of desperation. He had awoken my sexuality that had been dormant for so many years after the death of my husband. He had, essentially, started the motor running and left - leaving me sexually frustrated. I still question what it is that is wrong with ME. My friends do their best to try and be jovial with me about the situation, to make me feel better, but he knew what he was doing from day one. My counselling is helping me to make sense of it. We did have a relationship, of sorts, and I think he did love me, but it has all brought my self-loathing issues back to square one. I can't help feeling used and I wonder how far he would have let it go. Would I have potentially lost my virginity to a gay man? I think back to other things over the course of the relationship that were unusual. He didn't like me learning Polish, which I was doing for him. He took a real exception to it. He also accused me of tempting him, sexually, which I was certainly not doing deliberately. The whole time, he had the ultimate control but he never stopped our intimacy and he initiated the kiss.

I can only think that he is an immature, twisted man who is more to be pitied than vilified. I was not going to wait around until he got his novelty of screwing a cripple, or whatever he was planning.

The important thing is, now, that I'm single and learning to love myself. I hope, by participating in this book, other people will realise the problems people with disabilities face with intimacy, and that we are not here to be used. Half of the battle with prejudice also comes from self-prejudice. If we can tackle these problems one at a time, who knows what disabled men and women can be capable of.

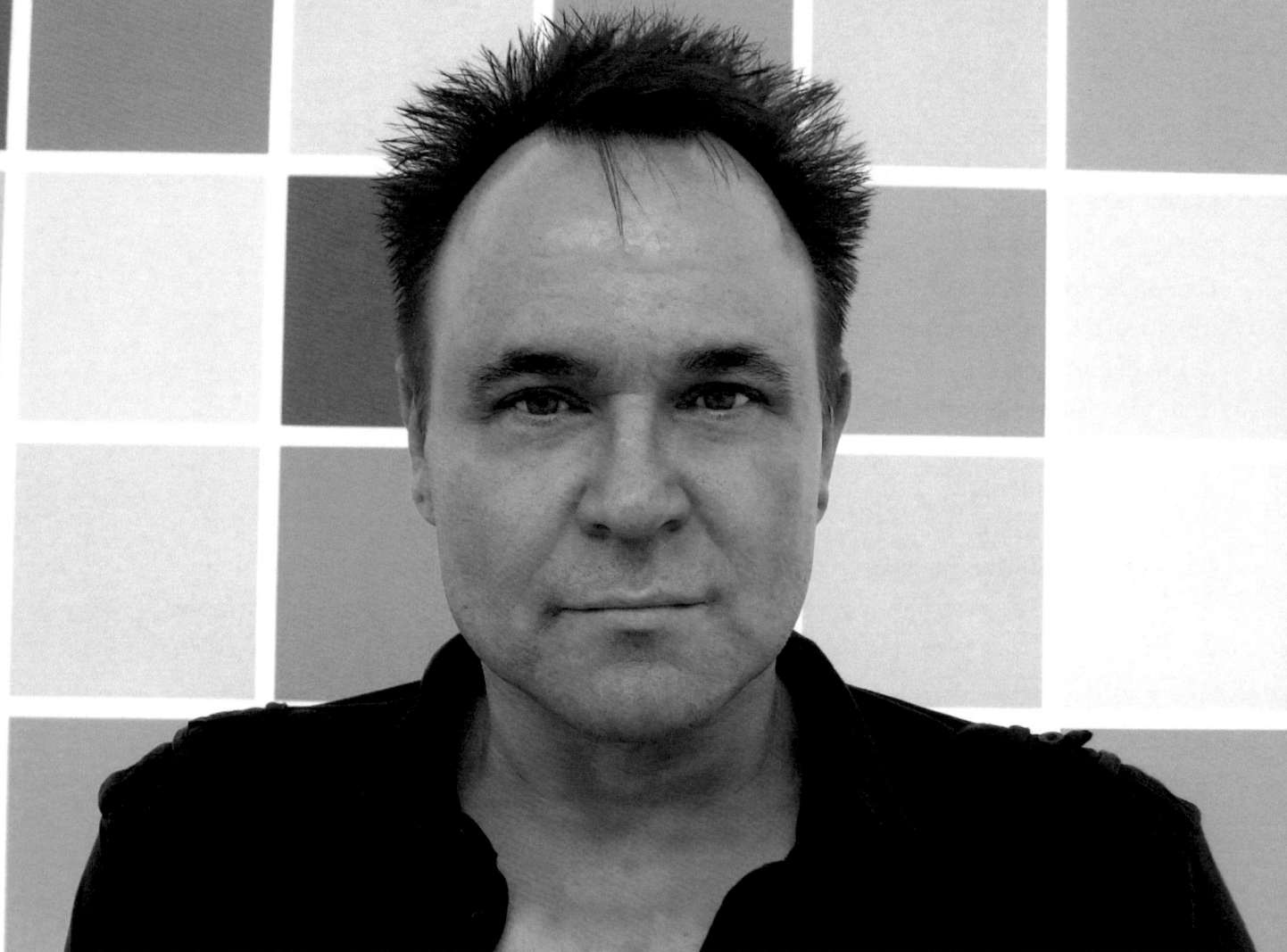

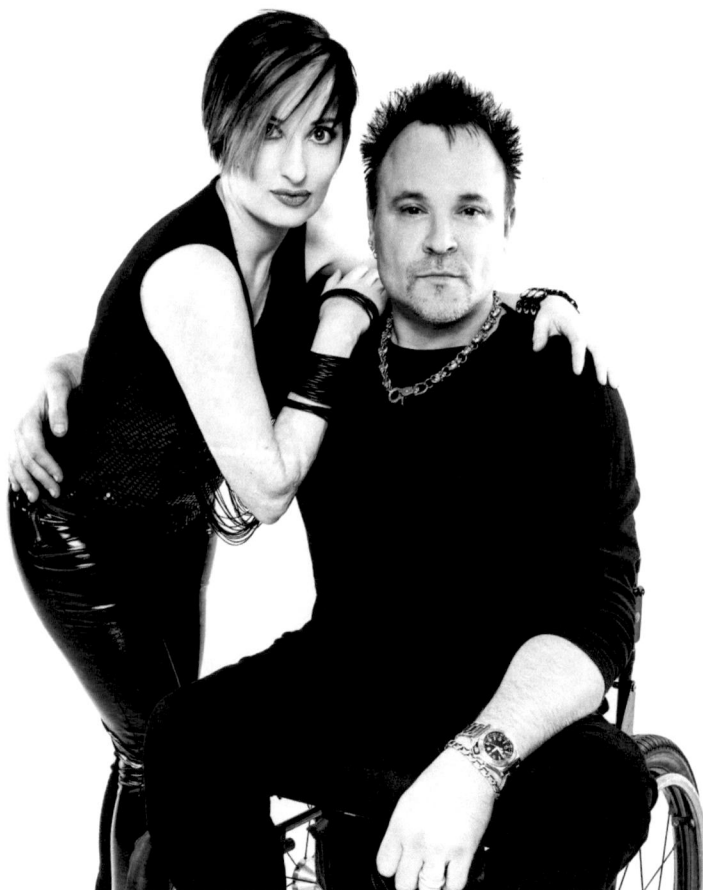

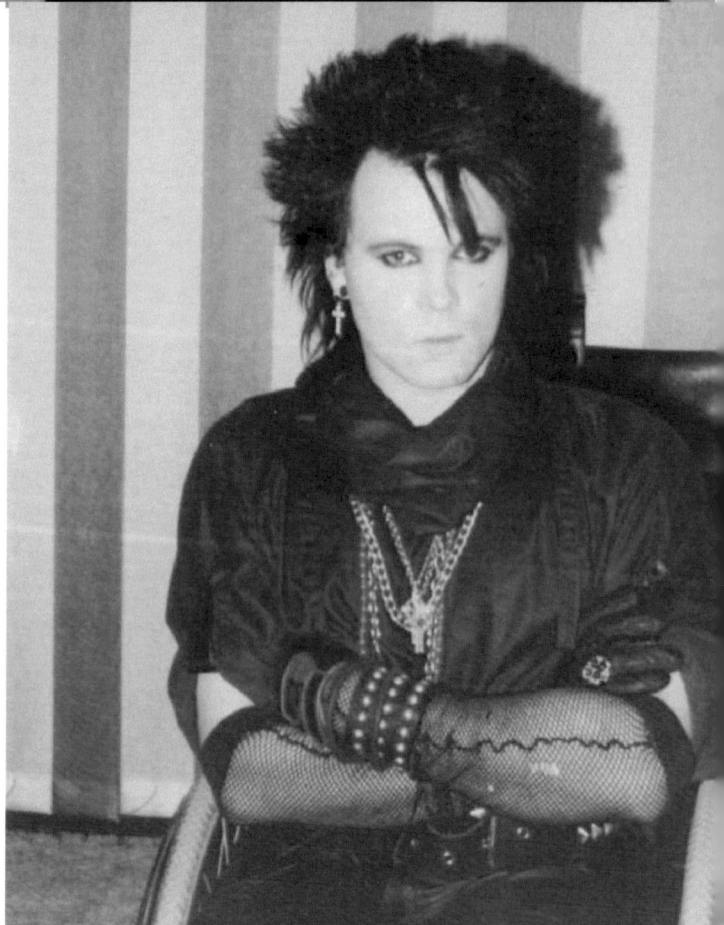

Mik Scarlet is a 49 year old journalist, broadcaster, musician and Equality Consultant who is also one half of our 'Love Lounge' team. He is married and lives in Camden, London.

Mik's story

To be honest, I get a little bored of talking about my sex life. As well as it being seen as a legitimate topic of conversation by most non-disabled people I meet, I also began my career in the media during the early 1990s working on "yoof" TV shows, where we talked about nothing but sex, and drugs and rock and roll, as well as love, body image and the rest of the stuff that eats away at your self confidence as a teenager. As well as being one of the presenting team, I fronted an entire documentary on the subject of sex and disability. That went out in 1991, which shows that this is a subject that has interested our society for decades... if not longer. But I don't want my chapter in this book to just be for the sordid interest of those who are desperate to ask, 'can you still do it in a wheelchair?' No. I want to explore my early experiences of the 'old in out' to give a deeper insight into what it is to be a sexual being and be disabled.

So what is my impairment? Well, it's a long and rather complicated story. I shall give you the short version as not to bore you to death.

I was born with a rare form of cancer called an Adrenal Neuroblastoma. There are only 100 cases per year worldwide, and even today it is very hard to cure. Back when I was born, in 1965, it was a death sentence. My parents were given a prognosis of about five days when I was first diagnosed, but my medical team insisted that they tried a new drug and surgical technique and, without anyone expecting it, I survived. Even after the original success I was only given five years to live. Yet, in 2015 I will be celebrating my Fiftieth birthday, and with no sign of any cancer returning during all those years (touch wood). As a child the treatment left me paralysed down my right side, from my waist down. So I wore a leg brace, or calliper as we called it back then, and I walked with a limp. I also wore a nappy as I could not control my bladder. Otherwise, I was just like all my non-disabled mates and, after some fighting by my parents, I ended up going to a mainstream school. I was the only disabled kid at my infants and juniors and I remember the girls liking me, as I was easy to catch in games of kiss chase. At least I put it down to that, but looking back at pictures of me at that time I think me being rather cute might also have helped! I think that this feeling that I was only picked as I was easy to catch, as the girls ran around our play ground in giggling gangs, fighting to kiss us boys, all of whom were disgusted by the very thought, highlights what it is to grow up with an impairment. Without knowing why, I just felt I wasn't attractive.

I wasn't allowed to play at being Steve Austin, the Six Million Dollar Man, when we played bionic man in the playground. Instead I had to be the six pence kid, the hero's sidekick, even though I really had a metal leg! I was also really bad at sport, which is how boys measure themselves from an early age. No one came out and said, "you aren't as good as us," but I felt that way. As I turned from a child into an angst-ridden teenager, I was sure that no girl would ever look at me, let alone have sex with me! But hope is a strong emotion. However, hope cannot conquer wearing a leg bag filled with your wee. I had moved up from a nappy to this awful brown rubber leg bag as I started at high school and I hated the thing. I couldn't change with the other boys when I tried to attempt sport, and so changed with the teachers (a whole other book there I must say). This set me further apart from my mates, but I easily blamed this on a fear that one of them might steal my leg brace for a laugh. It is something you learn to be brilliant at when you are incontinent at a mainstream school; lying your tits off. In fact it set me up to be a superb liar in adulthood, and the only person who can tell when I'm lying, instantly, is my wife. Apparently I get a look and it's a dead give away, although no one else has ever spotted this look. Sorry, I'm getting ahead of myself here. Wife? I'm still a virgin at this point and was sure I would remain that way forever.

During the summer of my 14th birthday, I decided to try to do something about this bag of piss strapped to the side of my leg. So instead of spending the six weeks of bliss away from school mucking about with my mates, I locked myself into my bedroom and tried to potty train myself. I spent day after day sat on a babies changing mat trying to control my bladder, while I enlarged my collection of Airfix models. By the end of the six weeks I was an expert in building, painting and detailing my models so they looked like those professional ones you see in model shops. I was also able to control my bladder. It transpired that when I was a baby my doctors told my Mum I would always be incontinent and so she didn't even try to train me not to pee myself. I cannot describe the sense of accomplishment that filled my growing frame as I returned to school that year. I could change with my schoolmates, and they didn't steal my calliper either. I also knew I could talk to girls, and they wouldn't notice the slight smell of wee. And I knew I could take my clothes off without the terror of explaining why I had all that awful brown rubber over my willy and why it had a bag of piss attached to it. I was reborn...and it was great.

This was when I discovered the music that would shape my life to come. Firstly, when we returned to school that year, our headmaster, Mr. Price, decided he needed to crush the dreams out of our working class minds and so gave us his 'think realistic' talk during one assembly. However, he walked on the stage with his dastardly plans ready to kill our dreams to Ian Dury's 'What A Waste.' He obviously had paid little attention to the lyrics, other than the list of possible jobs Mr. Dury turned down to be a musician. But for me this song changed my life. Until then I had no dreams, other than a sensible job in a factory... if I was lucky. But as I sat there I realised that Ian Dury was disabled and he was a popstar. I was disabled too, therefore I could also be a popstar. In an instant, a new Michael emerged; interested in fashion and music... and rebellion. Following quickly on this moment of epiphany came another, even more important one: I discovered Gary Numan. Yes, the robot king of synth pop stirred something in me that shaped the rest of my life. I joined a band, playing keyboards, started dressing in black and wearing eyeliner but, most importantly, I became fascinating to the girls in my school. I really went for the whole human/robot thing that was Gary Numan's early image, and the girls loved it. Almost overnight, I went from the shy nerdy kid who couldn't talk to girls to the weird, fashionable dude who didn't talk to girls because he was so cool. I don't envy kids today, who have to be all loud and brash. I had it made. My shyness was now a boon, and girls fought to get a few words out of me. Having said all that, I still couldn't believe that they might fancy me. I mean I was the disabled kid. I walked with a limp! I can look back at this point in my life and laugh, as I now know how many of those girls I called my friends were desperate to call me boyfriend. Eventually, I met one girl who was so forward not even I could fail to understand her intentions, and I found myself one of a couple for the first time.

On the way to this wonderful position I should note I had a few disasters. The worst one occurred the night I slow danced with the wonderful Tina Price. I had such a crush on this vision of teenage perfection I am amazed my heart still beat in her presence. We had become firm friends, however, and she was always telling me how funny I was, and that I was a great bloke. Sadly Tina had a thing for guys who were not great blokes, otherwise known as bastards, and so I was absolutely sure she would never go for me. Then one night, at a school disco, she asked me to dance…to a slowie. Was this my chance?

As we rubbed our teenage bodies against each other, she suddenly let out a deafening shriek. I had placed my paralysed foot on hers, and the added weight of my metal calliper had caused me to break her toe. The total horror! As I took her weight, and helped her to limp home that night, I knew my chance had passed and went back to being just a mate. Many years later she scolded me for this idea, as she thought I was amazing too, and was always sad that it never happened between us. I only mention it as I think it shows how the littlest thing can damage your confidence at that age, disabled or not. I should also point out that she didn't tell me how she felt either. Girls at that age do seem to think boys should be mind readers. Don't wait. If you fancy someone tell them. Anyway, after the Tina incident I avoided slow dancing and made sure I never seriously injured my now new girlfriend. As 1981 began I felt on top of the world. That'll teach me.

On the morning of my German O Level exam I awoke to find myself in loads of pain and finding it hard to stand. My mum, thinking I was faking it I imagine, called a cab and I was sent off to school. On arrival I collapsed, an ambulance was called and I was soon in hospital. Typically, my school sent a teacher to sit with me in the ward so I could take the exam. Shortly after, it was discovered that my spine had collapsed as a side effect of my cancer treatment as a baby. I then spent six months in hospital undergoing surgery. It was a weird experience. At first I was put in a terminal ward, as everyone was sure my cancer had returned. I spent two months in a ward where everyone else died. At one point I was told, by mistake, I was also dying. As I lay there,

Mik's story

trying to pluck up the courage to ring my Mum to tell her the awful news, I listed all the things I would never do. I would never dye my hair, never go clubbing, never travel and, yes, never have sex. I promised myself that if I got through this I would never be that shy idiot who never asked out the girls he fancied. I would live for today and actually do stuff, instead of dreaming about it.

I was then transferred to another hospital, to have yet more surgery. This one went a bit wrong and I got an infection that should have killed me. As I lay in my bed, with green smelly stuff oozing from my operation scars, my girlfriend came to see me. She lasted about five minutes and I never saw her again. I never held it against her. She was a teenager too, and this was some heavy shit to contend with at any age. Anyway, I had to focus on not dying, so I forgot sex and all that stuff. There was another kid who was sixteen, two beds over from mine. Every morning when it was time to get washed, he would go all red. After the curtains were pulled back and we were all sweet smelling and clean, he would be even redder. None of us could understand why, and then one morning it all became clear.

On this morning, I found myself being washed by one of the student nurses. Children's wards are always the favourite haunt of student nurses, as the kids are so sweet and not much trouble. This nurse was one, even the younger kids had recognised, as being way too attractive to be a nurse. Model or popstar maybe, but a nurse? As she closed the curtain, my heart raced and I instantly understood why my ward mate got so flustered when it was wash time. This nurse always was assigned this boy, and now it was my turn. As any teenage boy knows, when you are in the company of a very attractive woman, your body reacts whether you want it to or not and mine did exactly that, as she soaked my body with a soapy flannel. Oh god, what do I do? As she washed the suds off, she looked at my now full erect member, smiled and said "I can't leave you like that, can I?" Suddenly I was in her mouth and bingo... my first orgasm, and it was not at my own hand. This then became a regular thing, and I now shared a knowing smile with the boy. At this point I was moved into a side ward, and things got even steamier. Then one day my parents came to visit me, pushed past the closed curtains only to find this nurse straddling me in the throes of sex. Without missing a beat, she jumped off me, and doing up her dress said to my open mouthed parents, "Michael's been telling me all about his life. Isn't he brave?" My Step Father laughed and said, "nice one son," and the incident was never mentioned again.

Shortly after this period of forbidden sex, I was taken off one of the drugs that were part of my treatment regime. Suddenly I lost the ability to achieve erections. The poor nurse could not really tell anyone, as this would involve admitting that she was having sex with at least two of the patients. So I had to pluck up the courage to raise it with my surgical team and, after a few checks, they announced it looked like the nerves that served the motor function of my penis had been trapped in scar tissue... and that I would never manage to get erect again! After finally tasting what sex was, I had it torn away from me, forever. To say I became depressed at this point is an understatement. When I was told I might never walk again, I really thought, "yes, no more PE." But this was different. This was sex. I had not only had to say goodbye to walking but to having sex. When I left hospital, all I wanted to do was die. I even tried it once, but stopped with seconds to go, as I didn't want my Mum to find my body. While I planned another way of taking my life, life changed and I got slowly better.

Once out of hospital, I found myself trapped at home. I was far too weak to wheel my own chair and had to rely on others to push me. I was stuck at home with no friends at all. Anyone who has experienced a major illness will agree, especially when you are so young, that all of your friends slowly disappear until you have none. This is something that really hurts, and makes you feel so very different from the person you once were. For me, this period was weird. I had been disabled, yet now I was more disabled. I had to learn how to do everything all over again. I even had to potty train myself again. Eventually I started to get stronger and could push myself a bit. As my health returned, I needed something to do. Luckily I had received a large cheque of back paid benefits (something to do with being turned down for them when I was twelve which turned out to be wrong) and so I "wisely" invested most of it in some musical equipment. A synth, a drum machine and a mixer, which allowed me to sit for hours teaching myself how to play.

I soon found I could bang out pretty close covers of almost the entire Human League 'Dare' album. I also started back at school, if only to re-sit the exams I missed, due to my rush into hospital. This allowed me to attend school out of uniform, and so I found myself cool again. I gained a small group of mates, mostly girls, and we swapped makeup tips. I should point out that by this time I was a hardened (if that is the right word) New Romantic, so I wore more make up than most of my female mates. I took a correspondence course on stage makeup and was soon in demand, getting my female friends ready for their nights out.

I could not begin to believe that any of these fancied me in any way. I mean, not only was I a wheelchair user but my cock did not work. No one would ever want to have sex with me! So I went down the 'straight gay mate' route. I was the best mate they could ever have. They told me their secrets, cried on my shoulder, and I advised them on what straight boys wanted. For a while it seemed great. But I wanted to be loved too. It occurred to me that if I couldn't have sex with a girl, I could with a boy. If I couldn't give, so to speak, I could still receive. One night I tried getting off with one of my gay mates, but it became very clear it was not for me. If for no other reason than the stubble... shudder. The scratchiness of the male face put me right off. No, I was definitely straight. ARSE! If the world of gayness was out, then what was I to do? Well, at the time, I hung round with a group of very active lesbian feminists, and one drunken night I told them of my predicament. After much laughter, they explained their mirth. They have sex with girls, and they DIDN'T HAVE A PENIS. If they could, they were pretty sure I could too. They also claimed that to them, who truly believed that every act of penetration was an act of rape (it was a radical time back then), I was the perfect man. I soon became a fixture on their rallies - the only male allowed. I also began hanging around with one member in particular and we became closest of mates.

Then one day she asked if I would visit her home and pretend to be her boyfriend. Her parents had been hassling her about her sexuality and she wanted to throw them off the scent, at least for a while. This all backfired, as when I finally turned up at her front door, her parents threw a real wobbly. They were horrified she was going out with a cripple, and listed all the reasons why I was such a bad choice to my face. I couldn't do the gardening, paint the ceiling or go up into the loft for a start, and then it got much more personal. Was she prepared for a life caring for me and facing the stigma of being with someone disabled? She obviously lost it and, before the row went nuclear, we left.

This attitude shocked us both to the core and also threw us together. Later that night we went from being mates, to being lovers. So that backfired, eh? I soon found that my lack of ability to get erect was no bar to having a wonderful sex life. In fact, it appeared to set me free from many of the biological rules of masculinity.

You see, while I had no motor function, or I couldn't get stiff, I had full sensation. So I could still feel everything. It transpires that without the mechanical bit of sex, a male sexuality is much more like a female's and it is possible to achieve multiple orgasms. Good huh? As I realised that my lack of function might actually be a route to an even more fulfilling sex life, I decided to read up on all things sex. I wanted to be an expert at everything, and so I knuckled down to some serious study of the subject. Books on everything from making love to your woman like a woman; through clinical studies of how the body worked during sexual excitement; to more extreme stuff, like manuals on torture, became my bedside reading. Alongside my now regular practical experience, I packed my little mind with all manner of knowledge about sex and sexuality, and I grew in my sexual confidence day by day. However, I still didn't feel attractive. My relationship was great, but I couldn't shake the feeling that we had been thrown together by forces other than attraction, and this ate away at me. Eventually I ended it and, from her heart broken reaction, I realised that it was much more than I had understood. To this day I feel guilty about that period, but as long as you learn from your regrets you become a better person. I hope!

Newly single I wanted to use my skills to rock the world of new partners. Sure this sounds a bit naff, but I was nineteen by this time and I felt I had so much to catch up on. I wanted to experience more. I won't bore you with a detailed description of my youthful exploits, but I will say that I soon found that my disability, and the way my body functioned sexually, were not a barrier to forming relationships or having sex. I would not say I truly shook the feeling that it would be though. So every time I entered a new relationship, I was terrified of telling my new partner what did and didn't work in the trouser department, despite only ever having one bad reaction. I had one girl rather upset, that I expected a reciprocal sexual relationship, as she was expecting me to pleasure her with no need for payback. I also had one girl ask if she could think about it. Instead of saying "OK," I finished with her on the spot. Overreaction maybe, but no one "thinks" about being with me.

I had two more long-term relationships before meeting my now wife. I won't deny that these two were not the happiest relationships, mainly as I allowed my confidence to be knocked by my ex-partners. I now see that they only did this in a vain attempt to keep me around, but at the time I felt like I just wasn't enough for them, both physically and as a person. When I split from them both, I was shocked at how upset they both were. If I was such an awful boyfriend, why the floods of tears? Sadly, I could not see that they were as wrecked with confidence issues as I was, and this manifested itself in a need to make me feel less confident. Luckily my wife Diane has no such issues, and it's one of the many reasons why I love her. She loves me, everything about me, and tells me so at every opportunity. I am a lucky son of a gun.

Before I go, I wanted to say that I now know how amazing love is. I used to believe this "you've got to work at it" myth, but in my experience if you feel like you are working at it then it's not love. If you have issues of confidence, this attitude that 'love is hard' makes you easy to manipulate. Love should be a walk in the park. Sure you might have to wrap up if it's cold, and you might need to stop for a coffee or a toilet break, but that's not the same as feeling like you need to build the park and do all the planting. It should be a pleasant enjoyable thing, not a slog. I know I am really lucky. I am now in the kind of relationship that I really didn't think existed. I not only live with my wife, but I work with her too. We are together 24 hours a day, seven days a week and we rarely raise our voices to each other. Why? - Because we really love each other. I only tell you this, as if I had known this kind of love existed in my past I would have left unhappy, unhealthy relationships much sooner. However, we are all the sum of our history so all of those unhappy relationships led me to be the person who Diane loves today, which means that, no matter how hard it was to be there at the time, I owe all of my ex-partners a debt of thanks. Without them, there would be no Diane and that would be the worst thing of all.

Don't let society tell you that because you are disabled, you aren't sexy or sexual. You are amazing and I know there is someone out there for everyone. You just need to be happy, to keep looking, never let the knockbacks damage your desire to find love, and see every experience as positive. Might sound like a cheap self-help book, but as I get older (50 next year) I see the truth in these words. It's the advice I wish I had got, back as a spotty teenager - that, and love who you see in the mirror.

Z's story

Over the last fifteen years, one of my major concerns has been the logistics of sex. Particularly a one night stand. I'm in a wheelchair, I need help to get dressed, and would also need help to get from the bed to my wheelchair then to the bathroom. So understandably, the thought of the 'after sex' situation filled me with anxiety.

Over time, I've had some experiences that have all proved to be ok, as I felt comfortable around the people I was with. However, I thought I'd share a story with you that happened to me recently that blew all my preconceived ideas, and worries, out of the water.

I just can't watch the John Lewis Christmas advert in the same way now. Oh, sorry I haven't mentioned that one of the protagonists of this story is in fact a penguin. Ok, a man dressed up as a penguin...which only made the story (and banter afterwards from my girl friends) even funnier.

So, it was a girls' weekend away...the rest of the girls were married with children. There were a few jokes about me pulling but that's never my first thought - I'm always just out for a good time singing and dancing - and don't expect to cop off with guys in a nightclub situation now that I'm in a wheelchair. It's just too much of a barrier, I find - they're less likely to pull me on a night out than a walking girl, as they're not likely to want to undertake the challenge and potential complexities of 'going back' with a woman in a wheelchair for just one night. That's how I've viewed it before anyway.

However, Mr. Penguin Man thought differently and seemed uber keen on me. And no, I wasn't dressed as a fish. We'd been talking all night and he was hilarious too (always a bonus in my book) and eventually we said about going back to the room.

Now my friends can be fairly protective of me at times - they'll tell guys to back off or not touch me because I used to be in a lot of pain so it genuinely was a problem years ago, when guys pulled me around on the dance floor, but now I may be like, "Er, I quite fancy him on me actually!" So the girls were worried if I'd be ok, and was I too drunk, and checking that they'd be able to hear me if I needed them. All of this was going on unbeknown to me...clucking hens!

I was sharing a room with a very good friend of mine. Already she was going to be in the bunkroom, a children's room within the main room, so it wasn't like I was chucking her out by bringing him back. She took me to the loo while he was waiting on the bed - we were all very drunk so it wasn't as awkward as it sounds, all chatting and laughing and music was on. I've got visions of you reading this and imagining him waiting for his woman to get on the bed and it all being very cold, awkward and clinical. It wasn't.

So, my friend says, what shall I do? Get you undressed and in your nightie?! I was cracking up thinking that would look so odd. Nope, he could undress me like in any normal situation.

So we had our night of, not the best fun I've ever had (!), whilst my friend had passed out drunk in the next room. She wasn't so keen on her mother hen duties at this point, and would have been no use to anyone.

When I spotted her going to the loo at 7am, I was also needing to go so called her in to get me up. Penguin was still asleep… I realised I was totally naked… awkward for me and my friend! My clothes had been chucked away from the bed, and the room was in pitch darkness. So it's only normal, surely, for your best mate to be crawling on her hands and knees searching for your knickers and a top amongst the strewn clothes and 80's fancy dress paraphernalia across the floor, whilst I lay there starkers with a now skinned penguin next to me. If only my knickers had also been neon pink, she may have had a better chance of finding them.

Mr. Penguin started to stir, as we were pretty much in hysterics right now! So my friend swiftly stood up, pretending she was only in the room to get a drink. He went to the bathroom and the frantic hunt for knickers continued. Back in commando position she triumphed and quickly got my top and pants on; he walks in and I'm ready. Phew. Seamless. Kind of.

It was such a good laugh meeting up with the other girls in the morning and sharing all the tales - I can't tell you the amount of jokes bouncing around. 'Friend must've found the knickers by them sticking to her elbow; lucky I can't walk else I'd be doing the penguin walk the morning after; Pingu.' Now the human parody of the John Lewis advert, I think, has actually been modelled on me.

All in all, it was a fun experience, and one that my friend and I felt bonded over and really pleased to have shared. How nice that I feel comfortable enough with my friends, and they with me, to share such an experience and it not be awkward. I'm so grateful for the support of my friends through all of my years of living with a chronic illness, and the fact we've remained so close. They know all of my anxieties about this topic, so it all just came together that night. As it were, ahem.

Now that this rather big barrier of having sex as a one night stand, and away from my home and normal support system etc, has occurred without a problem, it has filled me with confidence to know that, as a wheelchair user, I can still have just as much fun. Men are up for taking a girl in a wheelchair in for a one night stand, and with humour (and a bit of empathy) it doesn't have to be an angst ridden experience. Alcohol obviously helped too...but that's the same for everyone on a night out isn't it?

Z's story

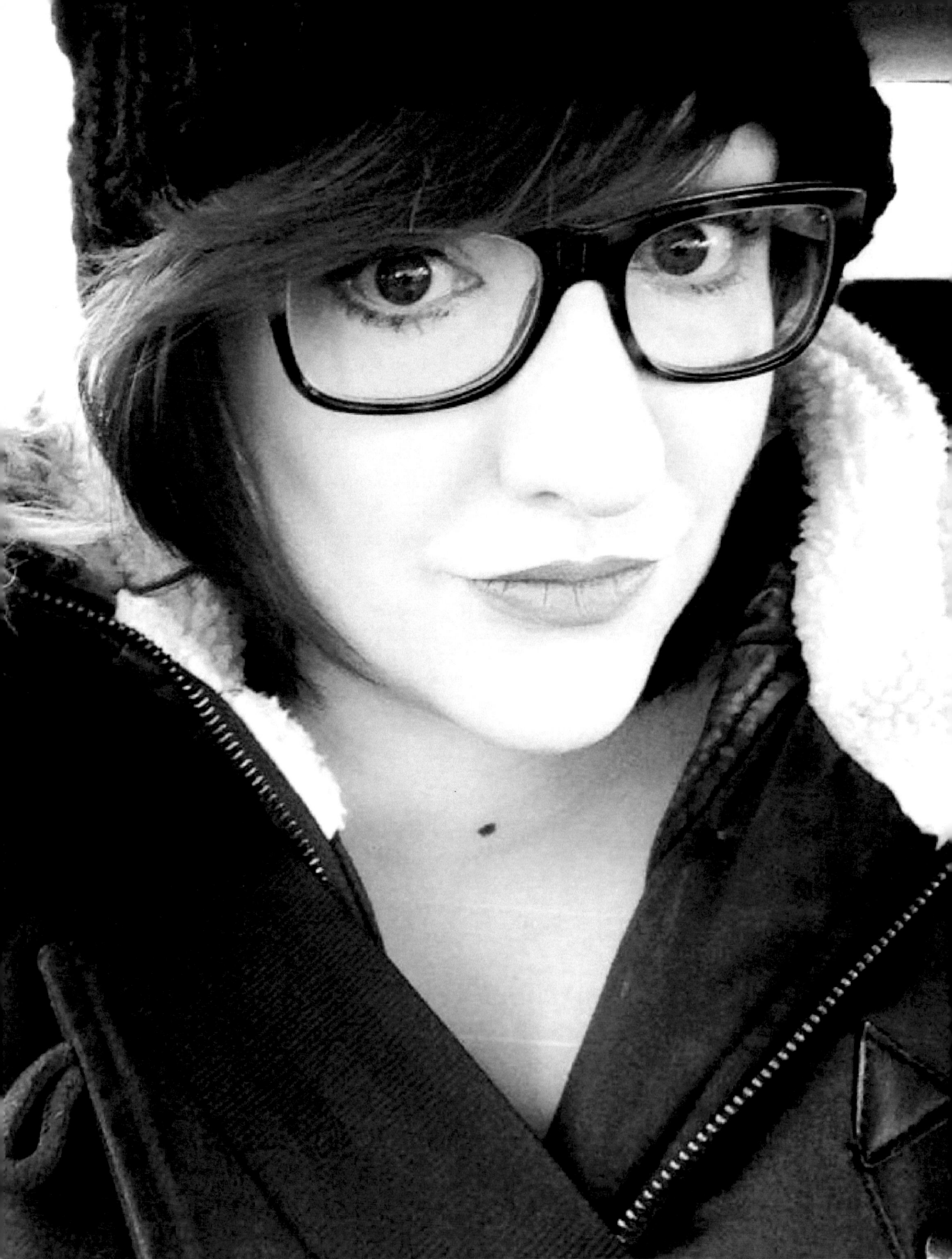

Sarah Willow is a 28 year old MA graduate and writer from Lancashire. She has a condition called Ehlers-Danlos Syndrome Type III, which means her joints hyper extend due to faulty collagen, leaving her in a lot of pain.

Sarah's story

Then

You know that shy, invisible kid from your form at school? No? You obviously don't, not many do. But I do, because I was that kid. The only few that acknowledged my existence were a group of dickheads that called me 'Peg Leg', and the bitch girls that ruined my high school life. Even after eighteen months of being home-schooled they didn't forget me. As soon as I returned in Year 10, there they were, with their smart-arse comments, making me want to throw myself under a bus. I didn't belong anywhere, certainly not here.

I wasn't even picked on for being disabled, I wasn't disabled; I was accident-prone, always on crutches or in a wheelchair, forever breaking a leg, an ankle, a hip. Yep, I broke my hip when I was thirteen, like a geriatric - and then 'Peg Leg' was born.

I left school at sixteen and something wasn't right. The physical pain in my back, knees, hips, was excruciating; it had been bad since my hip operation (aged 13) but it was getting worse. I've never been one to cry in pain, my threshold has always been quite high, but this pain, this new agonising pain was causing me to scream, even with the slightest movement. My friends all went off to college and then university, and I was either so tired I could barely speak, or high off my face on morphine (it was prescribed, don't panic). I saw my GP, God knows how many times, had every test under the sun, and then referred to orthopaedics, rheumatologists, physiotherapists and finally, psychiatrists. I was told that the pain was 'all in my head,' and I was manifesting the lack of relationship I had with my dad into physical pain. After being told that I was 'making it up,' for years, I began to question whether I was.

My only real solace was the internet, and luckily I came from a generation before Facebook and during the days of MSN Messenger and MySpace; I'd sit at my computer talking to random strangers online. They didn't know my problems, they didn't know I was the girl that didn't belong anywhere. Online, I could be anyone. I only usually lied about my age and sometimes where I was from; or depending on how fit they were, if I had a boyfriend.

I met Tony in a chat room a few months before my eighteenth birthday, I didn't lie to him. He was twenty-one, 6'5" and a bassist in a band. Tick, tick, tick. Oh, and he was fucking gorgeous; like beautiful. He was the clichéd tall, dark and handsome. I hate that word, handsome always sounds like something my mum would say. He was hot. We chatted every day and night for weeks, online, via text, on the phone. His desktop background was a picture of me; it's pathetic now, when you think about it, but as a 17 year old, I found it adorable.

I was shitting myself. How did I tell him that I was mental? 'Oh, by the way, I fake pain because I miss my dad. I'm that tapped, I use crutches and sometimes a wheelchair, but don't worry, as soon as I get in touch with my dad the pain will go away, and I'll be normal.' Yeah, that sounded insane. He'd run a bloody mile. So, I did what any teenage girl would do, and I didn't mention it.

We eventually met, after seven weeks of constant chatting. He picked me up and took me for dinner. I'd heard so many horror stories of people faking their profile pictures, but that didn't happen; Tony was Tony. 6'5" and oh my days, fit. He was really nervous; I was shaking and talked so much during the car ride that my jaw hurt. To impress him I wore the lowest-cut top I had, a skirt and the most ridiculous knee-high stiletto boots (which I still question to this day). He parked miles away from the restaurant and I panicked, when I say miles away, it was probably about a 5 minute walk but it was still too far for my crippled, stupid body. I didn't want to ask him to park closer in case he thought I was a lazy bitch but I also didn't want to have that agonising walk, as I couldn't exactly pop some pills whilst he was sat in front of me. We stayed in the car for an hour and talked, but it was constantly in the back of my mind that we needed to get out and hike for food. When we finally made it to the restaurant I excused myself, stuck my head under the tap in the toilets and swallowed a mouthful of painkillers, stretched my back, checked myself in the mirror, and went back to him with a huge smile on my face. My boobs looked great, my hair looked great and I felt like shit – he had no idea. We got on really well and I knew he liked me as much as I liked him.

He asked me to be his girlfriend a week later and, obviously, I agreed. He lived half an hour away but came to my house every night ,when he finished work, and stayed over at weekends. When we met he was a virgin; I wasn't. I was incredibly shy; he wasn't. He was adventurous, he wanted us to do everything, we had sex in his car, in fields, on a train, we role-played, we watched porn; I did anything he wanted. I was madly in love with him. He was everything I ever wanted in a boyfriend; a musician, funny, sexy, tall, intelligent, cheeky and my family loved him; he had to eventually find out that I'd lost the plot and I was dreading that day. He knew I'd had a hip operation and I told him I took tablets because it still hurt.

A few weeks into our relationship I had a really bad flare-up and had to explain to him the pain I was constantly in. I was petrified that he was going to get in his car, never to return again but he took it really well, or as well as he could have, he didn't leg it, he seemed sad that I hadn't told him sooner.

The pain was so intense that I couldn't walk, and spent three weeks in bed. I somehow managed to open my legs enough for my boyfriend to fuck me each night he visited me. He'd go home around 10pm and I'd still be awake until 5am paying for all the thrusting with pain. After a few nights I told him it was hurting to have sex. He apologised profusely, kissed me and got in bed for a cuddle. I lay with my head on his chest; falling asleep (I hadn't slept properly in weeks), he was watching telly and then slowly his hand moved up my shirt and stopped at my bra, I pretended to sleep, then his hand moved inside my bra. I couldn't fucking believe it, I'd just told him how much pain I was in and he still wanted to get his leg over. I jokingly told him to stop, I was tired and he got up and left, if I was tired, he'd go so I could sleep. I knew he was pissed off. I cried all night. I couldn't lose him. I needed to sort my head out; I needed this pain to disappear.

He came to see me the next night and didn't try anything. The night after that I felt guilty, I didn't really understand how difficult it was for him to see me like this and, as sex was such a huge part of our relationship, I couldn't deny him that. I looked and felt like shit but awkwardly shuffled down the bed and began giving him a blowjob. I'm a fan of oral sex, always have been, but I really wasn't into it this night, maybe because I felt like I was being stabbed repeatedly in my knees and back. Anyway, I was there doing my 'job' being an amazing girlfriend, and I heard the loudest crack, I felt like my eardrum had burst and someone had hit me in the face with a brick. Tony tried to sit up but I frantically pushed him back down because I couldn't move. My jaw had dislocated and I was crying with a penis in my mouth. I had no idea how I was going to get out of this situation, I had my boyfriend asking me ridiculous questions that I couldn't answer because HIS DICK WAS STUCK IN MY MOUTH and I was terrified that my mother was going to walk in on us and have to manually remove me from his groin. He wriggled for what seemed like a year, but in reality was a few seconds, and then nature helped - as having a crying girl attached to your penis isn't much of a turn on. This dislocation business had only happened once before: when I was eating my tea, I bit into whatever I was eating and my jaw popped out, it was crippling but somehow rectified itself. I managed to detach myself from my boyfriend but my jaw was still out of place, my whole face was throbbing, my ears buzzed and I rubbed the sides of my face, willing it to go back in. It eventually did and I had a killer headache, face-ache and ear-ache all night. I couldn't look at Tony, I was so embarrassed. He was definitely going to leave me after this. I sat on the edge of the bed, hurting, sobbing, and hating myself with my back to him. He altered his position, put his legs either side of me, wrapped his arms around my waist and told me to stop panicking, because he loved me. In that moment (and I remember it well), I finally felt like I belonged somewhere.

Over the next year, I had a lot of flare-ups, my mum kicked off at my GP and he agreed that I wouldn't be seeing any more psychiatrists. I was depressed; I became a person that I didn't like; there was something wrong with me; we just didn't know what it was. Tony was the only person that cheered me up. He'd do something silly to make me laugh, or hold me so tight that nothing in the world could harm us, and only when I was with him, in our bubble, did I believe that things might get better. But

Sarah's story

Undressing Disability 123

when he went home, when I was alone in my room, the overthinking started ,and the mental torture I unleashed on myself commenced. How could things get better when there was nothing wrong? You can't get better if you're well.

Writing was the only way I expressed myself. In poetry, I could spill my deepest, darkest secrets from a pen, and twist these tormenting, melancholic feelings into something moving, perceptive, insightful. Like my idol Sylvia Plath, I too was 'terrified of this dark thing that sleeps in me.' I was scared that I was insane, that I might harm myself; that I'd lose myself to the darkness.

This night will be forever embedded into my mind; I can see it as clearly as if it happened yesterday…I picked up my pen to write, it was around 2am, the time I usually wrote how shit I felt. I wrote seven words and I dropped the pen in absolute agony. My hand ceased up, my fingers wouldn't move, my wrist ached. I reached for the pen but I couldn't hold it, and I sobbed. I was living with my grandparents at the time and I went to my Nan, (she was a night owl too) and cried. If I couldn't write, what could I do? How could I be a writer if I couldn't hold a fucking pen? I told Tony the next day and he dismissed it, telling me to use my laptop. I saved everything to my laptop anyway, but I liked to write poetry by hand so I could scribble all over the page, change sentences, add words - that was my process - and yet I was no longer able to do it that way. I kept trying to write but I got a few words in and my hand stopped working. The pain it caused wasn't worth it. I shrank further into my hole; I could barely see any light.

Tony took me out that weekend to cheer me up; we went to a restaurant and then had drinks in town. We sat in the corner of a dark bar; he sat me on his knee and asked me to go on holiday with him that summer. Two weeks alone with him was all I needed. I was back on crutches, my knees kept giving out and I was very unstable on my feet. I was a limping disaster. Eighteen and not able to function without a handful of drugs, wrist splints, knee braces, crutches – I hated this.

We went to the cinema; he parked quite close to the entrance, locked the car and practically ran towards the doors. I caught up eventually and had a go at him because he didn't wait for me, 'my legs are longer than yours, short-arse.' I'm 5'3" so there was a significant height difference between us, I didn't hold it against him. He seemed to always walk a lot faster when I was on crutches but I guess I was much slower, I probably just couldn't keep up with him. I never went out in my wheelchair with him because it was embarrassing - what teenage girl wants her boyfriend pushing her around? I didn't want him to have to deal with that so I'd struggle on my crutches or leave them behind and hold onto him. He preferred it when I was free of my walking aids, we looked normal, he didn't run off, he stayed by my side. That's all I wanted. It was making me worse though. Every time I went out with him and walked for more than a few minutes. The night would come and I'd consider the best way of chopping my legs off. I couldn't do it with a knife because I couldn't hold onto it and I didn't have enough force as my wrists and shoulders were screwed. I'd have to get my brother to do it. I'd sit up all night counting the hours until my next lot of painkillers, gripped by painsomnia, telling myself over and over again not to compromise, to know my limitations…but I'd do the same the week after.

The beginning of May, 2006, my mum and step-dad were furious with how I was being drugged up but nobody knew what was wrong with me. I was referred to rheumatology again, I had to wait 6 weeks for an appointment, but my step-dad called the hospital and asked when I could be seen if he paid. They gave me an appointment for three days later. My parents paid £300 for a five minute consultation. The consultant asked about my medical history, about my pain, how often it was happening, and examined me. He had me bending all over the place like a bloody contortionist. 'Little fingers at ninety degrees, thumbs bend to touch wrists, elbows hyperextend, as do knees, knees straight and palms of the hands flat on the floor.' What the hell was he doing? I know I'm flexible, I've heard all the jokes. I sat on the edge of the examination bed staring at my mum as the doctor made notes. He turned to me and told me that my pain was real and that I had Ehlers-Danlos Syndrome Type III. I wasn't mental. I wasn't making it up. I could have kissed him when he told me that something was wrong. I had a condition. I hadn't been lying for six years. EDS means I hyperextend due to faulty collagen. Each time I take a step my knee doesn't stop in the straight-position, it bends backwards and is damaging the joints, muscles, tendons, ligaments and skin, and this is happening throughout my body. He told me about the possibility of dislocations and how important physiotherapy and pain management were.

I was taken into hospital the week after, for intensive physio. Tony came to visit me every night for a week. It was obvious he was uncomfortable but I hated seeing people I loved suffering too. My best friend came to see me the second night and brought a balloon, cards and chocolates. The old lady in the next bed commented on how well we suited and how much he must love me, which he did, but my best mate very much preferred boys. I had loads of visitors, they all brought cards and gifts to cheer me up but Tony never did. My mum asked me about it one night and I hadn't even realised. He did work all day and come straight to the hospital though, he hardly had any time. Our holiday was booked for the week after I came out of hospital and I was dreading it. I wasn't up to going away, I was in so much pain, and the train ride to Torquay was six hours. I can hardly sit for ten minutes, never mind hours. We were going with his mum and dad; he dropped that on me a few weeks after he'd asked me. His mum was a snotty cow, she babied him and it made me sick. If I knew we were going with them I wouldn't have agreed.

We'd been together eighteen months by the time the holiday came and, a few nights before, I complained to my Nan about my concerns. I wasn't well enough; I could barely walk; I wanted to stay at home. But I didn't want to let him down. I wanted to be with him. My Nan called Tony's mum and begged her to look after me, she told her how ill I was and how well I hid the pain. His mum assured my Nan that she'd keep an eye on me and that we'd have a great time.

The train journey was horrendous. My shoulders ached, my knees killed, my hips were on fire; I hated every second of it. When we finally got to the complex, it was lovely, so peaceful with great views, but in the middle of nowhere. We had to walk half an hour to the nearest town and it was all downhill. You know what that means? Coming home was uphill. Holy shit, I wished I was dead after we walked back from having tea in town that night. I was up all night suffering. Tony was fast asleep next to me, pushing me away every time I tried to whisper to him. I needed a cuddle, some support, a fucking word of encouragement, but all I heard was snores. I needed him to wake up; I couldn't handle this pain alone. I texted my mum at about 2am, she called me right away and I sobbed down the phone to her. I couldn't move; the pain was excruciating; I felt alone; I didn't belong here.

Everyone was up at 7am, I hadn't been to sleep. Tony told me I was being dramatic and just needed to take some meds. I'd been popping pills all night and they didn't do a bloody thing, but he wouldn't know as he was sleeping like a baby. My mum called his mum and she said I'd be fine after I relaxed because she clearly knew more about my condition than I did. She also told my mum that I was being unfair and that Tony needed a holiday after all the time he spent working. Unfair? Fucking unfair? Was she having a laugh? I was being unfair? Wasn't I the one who spent the whole night crying her eyes out? Of course I was being unfair. I asked him to take me home and his mum lost it and started screaming at me for being selfish and ungrateful. I went into our bedroom, cried some more and called my mum. She was at Wigan train station half an hour later with my step-dad, coming to pick me up.

I pleaded with Tony to come with me, if I could have got on my knees, I would have. I wanted him to come home with me. I knew I needed to go back into hospital as the pain I was experiencing would only be controlled by a concoction of the good stuff. But I wanted him to come too; I needed him to support me.

I got dressed and put my pyjamas, and anything I'd unpacked, back in my suitcase. My parents were going to be six hours but I didn't want to be anywhere near his mother. I'd rather sit in the street. I hobbled out on my crutches. Tony took my suitcase and we waited for a taxi. When it finally came, he helped me in, kissed my forehead and half-waved as I was driven away.

Five hours I sat alone at that station, looking like an idiot, red-faced, snotty-nosed, heartbroken. Mum rang me so many times, 'he isn't worth it', 'what type of man leaves his disabled girlfriend in the middle of nowhere?' 'He's a piece of shit,' 'His mother is an evil bitch. If I ever get my hands on her…' My parents are incredible, they got off the train, hugged the life out of me, slagged Tony off ,and all three of us got straight on another train to take us up north. That journey home was worse than the one there, I'd had my heart ripped out of my chest. I'd rather dislocate every bone in my body repeatedly than feel like that.

I never heard from him again. He didn't contact me. He blocked me on every social media platform. He had his friends block me. What did I do wrong? I loved him. I loved him so much that he destroyed me.

I realised later that he was ashamed to be seen with me when I was using my splints or crutches. I think I knew it at the time but made excuses for him because I didn't want it to be true. Sometimes loving blindly is very dangerous.

Now

Ten years later – guess what? I'm still in agony. I still push my limitations and I hate accepting help. The only difference is I have an incredible boyfriend. He is so supportive, so caring and loving. He sits up with me of a night when I'm feeling shit, he rubs my legs when they're sore, he makes me hot water bottles, he pushes my wheelchair (even though I shout at him for crashing into things). Ian is the best thing that has ever happened to me, and he completely accepts my disability. He does everything in his power to help me and he doesn't realise how thankful I am for everything he does. I love him with all that I am. I belong with him.

A's story

After falling ill 8 years ago, from a rare illness, which has left me paralysed from the waist down, my sexual confidence has waned. I would definitely say I had an extremely high libido prior to my illness, and this completely vanished.

I went from a 10 stone fit, toned woman to a 17.5 stone marshmallow, wobbly bellied, and libido lost lady. The first time my other half and I even tried anything close to sex was about 2 years after I fell ill, after a boozed fuelled night of cocktails and shots! Needless to say it was not that successful, as I felt like a mannequin with no feeling or motions down in the fru fru, and couldn't have much appreciation or enjoyment of what was going on. This therefore left me feeling low and useless, as I could not feel what I had before for the man that I loved, and felt I could not give him what he wanted or needed.

These feelings only made me feel determined, and once I was off the steroids I would try to lose the weight and get things a little more back on track, and as normal for us both as possible. I needed to feel less wobbly and more attractive again. But I was doing this for me. Although my partner still thought I was beautiful, I felt that I needed to have confidence and feel comfortable in myself, to make things work properly and enjoy that part of our relationship once again…

I started to work hard on losing the wobble, and it slowly started to come off. My confidence was lifted, and this helped to improve my libido. Ok, so when having sex, it still did not give me much feeling, but the thought of what was going on was a turn on: the mind is a brilliant thing!!

'50 Shades of Grey' is not necessarily the best-written book in the world, but it definitely came along at the right time to get the imagination going. So there was not really any hard core S&M, but it certainly helped with positions that could be used, ways to stimulate each other and push the boundaries, to help us enjoy each other and remind us of how it used to be.

Do not be perturbed by falling off the bed, peeing slightly during (a weak bladder is not the most sexiest of things but sometimes you have to just go with these things), or by the lack of feeling when starting to explore again, I just tried and tried again. My feeling is still limited, but it is definitely more active than it initially was. If there's anything you can think of doing, and are comfortable to try, then do it. It is vital to build confidence, and for a woman to feel empowered. Make sure everything is trimmed and tamed…no stubble or monstrosities down there! Be comfortable with yourself, and this will build the confidence in the bedroom!

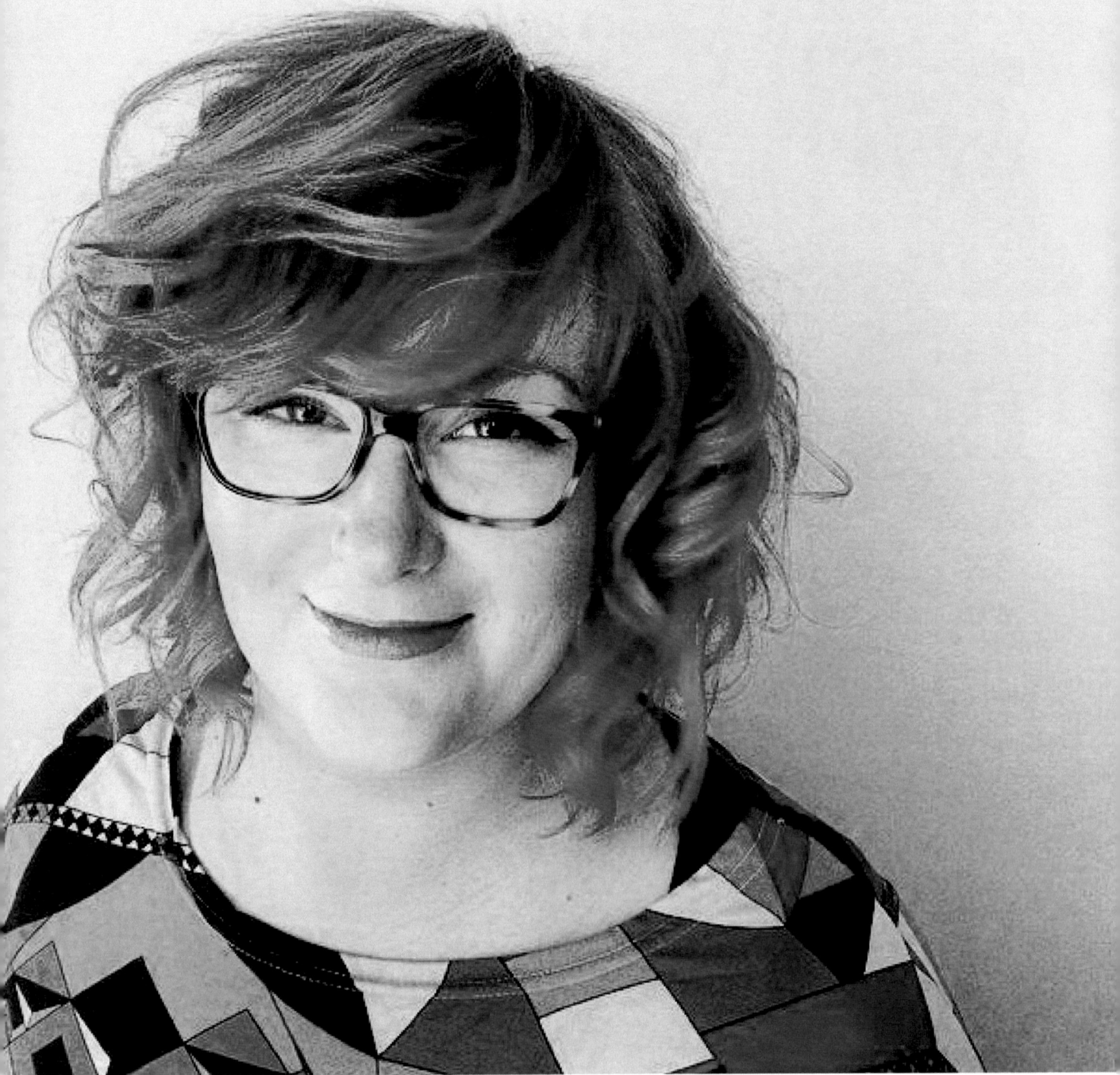

Emily Yates is a 24 year old accessibility consultant, accessible travel writer , blogger and presenter, currently based between London and Leeds.

She is studying for a Masters Degree in Disability Studies, from the University of Leeds, after graduating from Queen Mary, University of London, with an undergraduate degree in English Literature.

Emily has cerebral palsy and is a permanent wheelchair user.

Emily's story

Journey

About a week before I lost my virginity, my twin sister and Auntie decided to show me the ropes. Number 3 had taken me for a long weekend away about a month before, to the most beautiful cottage in the Peak District, but sex certainly wasn't on the cards after I'd rolled off the bed, hit my head on the bedside table and then decided to comfort myself by eating cereal and squirty cream for tea. Needless to say, we hadn't bought the cream with the intention of using it to distract me from my newly swollen forehead and dented pride…

We were in my Auntie's spare bedroom and I was having a bit of an 'oh-my-god-what-should-i-even-do-i-don't-know-how-to-have-sex' moment of sheer panic and desperation. I then asked them for advice. All too eager, the advice session turned into a hands-on position guide. We ended up having an afternoon full of giggles and guffaws as we practised straddling each other. It didn't particularly prepare me for what was to come, but I have a feeling the afternoon will be bared to all in great detail if I ever get married!

The day I properly met Number 3, we were on a boat, sea-lion watching in southern Africa. Both 16, we'd been selected to go on a journey of a lifetime. I was nominated because of my physical disability, and he'd previously had a brain tumour. I was sat on the central pillar on the boat, my legs dangling and my eyes scanning the water. He strode over and sat down. 'Do you want to put your legs on mine?' he asked, smiling. He lifted them up, rested them on his, and we talked and laughed the day away. Every morning, two separate registers were read out to correspond with the two trucks we were to travel in, and they changed daily, to make sure we all mingled. I vividly remember silently hoping that we'd be put together every single morning, not because I particularly fancied him, but because there was something about him that absolutely fascinated me in the weirdest way. I wanted to know more and more about him, to find out what made him tick and what he really loved. Very quickly, we had little 'in' jokes and I considered him a close friend.

There were so many star-filled nights that we sat together and chatted, recounting the day's events as he wrote them in his journal. Nothing romantic happened until years later; we were both with other people at this time and so desperate to make the most of the trip and not just each other. Even so, I knew I'd met someone that I wouldn't forget in a hurry.

Friend Zone

Before 16 and my journey of a lifetime, life had felt quite different for me. I was focused on two things: getting good grades at school and being one of the boys. My childhood heroes were Batman and Sporty Spice, whilst my sister loved Tinkerbell and Pocahontas (guess who always had to be John Smith?!) From a young age, I was always the best friend and football goalie rather than the love interest, but I absolutely adored that. Adored it, until my sudden boy attraction slapped me across the face and there was sweet fuck all I could do about it, having cemented myself into this little punky tomboy role that had previously suited me just fine.

There were a couple of boys I really fancied at school and strangely enough, the fact that I used a wheelchair never put me off being quite forward and asking them out. However, no amount of ballsy confidence could change their answers: 'oh Em, I like you, really I do, but I just value our friendship too much, let's not make this awkward, yeah?' And honestly, even though I was always disappointed, a little voice in my head always reminded me that these people actually really did like it when I was around, and the fact that they weren't jumping over each other to snog my face off was okay, and at least they were jumping over each other to sit next to me in class, so I could give them all the answers whilst talking about our favourite music, and how I'd put a good word in for them to that girl that they really liked.... Meanwhile, my sister was absolutely killing it in the boyfriend stakes, but she's always been the fit one.

The Big Change
After I returned from my African adventure at almost 17, this whirlwind world of independence seemed to unleash itself around me. Yes, I had Cerebral Palsy, but I'd been to Africa! Nothing could stop me and my close family, as always, pushed me to challenge myself at every opportunity. I can't express how lucky I was, and still am, to have such encouraging adults in my life.

From the age of 12, I'd played wheelchair basketball at club and county level. Although it has never been something I particularly excelled at, it provided great opportunities to meet others with disabilities and start conversations based on common interests and experiences. I'd briefly said hi to Number 1 a couple of times during tournaments when I was 16. I then started chatting to him online. He was from the South and a few years older than me, studying at University. We quickly got close and would be in contact every night. He was also a wheelchair user, and suddenly I wasn't even considering our disabilities, only how well we got on. I really liked this guy.

I remember going on my first ever five hour train journey, to stay with him and his family. I was a bag of nerves. Was it going to be the same in person? Was I going to fancy him as much? What if his parents didn't like me? Luckily, he was pretty nervous too, and we managed to laugh it off. His parents welcomed me with open arms and that was the start of a wonderful relationship. From then on, I'd save up as much money as possible to get the train down to see him for the weekend, as often as I could. I slowly got less nervous and more excited, and we just had a ridiculous amount of fun each time we were together. Yes, practicalities were sometimes tough: hauling both wheelchairs into his car must've done his head in from time to time, but not once did he complain. I was then accepted to study, at University in London, and we saw each other most weeks, which was great. I had some of my first sexual experiences with Number one, and although we never had sex in the penetrative sense, he made me realise that there was so much sexual fun to be had without it, and that this fun is even more exciting when you really, really appreciate the person that you're experiencing it with.

Things kind of fell apart when I moved to Australia for a year, as part of my degree. We'd been pulling in different directions and had been in an on-off relationship for a while, and that was the icing on the cake. Looking back now, it all seems like such a long time ago, and I can now see how young I was. It all felt so serious and yet it was so much fun. Even now, I don't have one bad word to say about Number 1. He was a true gent and the perfect first proper boyfriend. I feel blessed to still be able to call him a friend.

Infatuation

During 'off' periods with Number 1, and before we got serious whilst I was at University, I had a few flings with both able-bodied and disabled guys - one in particular, that taught me a lot of life lessons in a very short space of time. I have a real tendency to let people in and give my all without even realising what I'm doing. Of course, it's then too late and I've fallen head over wheels far too quickly with no way to get myself out again. I was absolutely infatuated with Number 2, and it was only ever going to end in tears.

It was a sports induced injury (relationship). He was gorgeous, muscly, older, and I looked forward to seeing him every week. He invited me over to his house one weekend, and that was it. I couldn't believe my luck. Me? With him? Good God, I had gone up in the world. The next few months were a blur of vodka and cokes and dressing in corsets so tight that my tits up at my neck would surely get me into the best metal clubs in town. Fortunately, he probably recognised that I had to practically pick my jaw up off the floor every time I saw him, and ended it before my heart was going to be anymore bruised. So, I was alone again and I STILL hadn't had sex. Jesus, things weren't going well. I felt pretty down at this point and it took me a while to man up and move on. But, it was nothing that a stint in Australia wouldn't sort out…

Oz

There's not much juicy gossip to share about my time in Australia from 2011-2012, which is why I think it's an important part of the story. For a whole year, I just focused on yours truly. I did what I wanted, when I wanted to do it, and it did me the world of good.

Whilst in Melbourne, I met A. She is still a massive part of my life now, and always will be. When I first arrived at my residential college, I saw this pretty girl with huge curly hair, who was also in a wheelchair. I was desperate to make friends, but she wasn't so sure at first. She told me later that she'd never wanted to associate herself with a 'disabled community' until she met me, but that quickly changed when we bought matching wheelchair love hoodies and booked plane tickets for a long weekend in Sydney. Just two wheelchair users, their bags, and loads of fun. What a huge success it was. The real cherry on top is the fact that, from being worried about our little trip to Sydney and how we'd manage, A travelled across the globe on her own to visit me and my family for Christmas in 2012. What an absolute babe.

Number 3

Something else happened whilst I was in Australia. Number 3, the guy that had fascinated me in Africa, got in contact. He was interested to know what I was doing out there and we agreed to Skype. As soon as we started talking, BAM! Something hit me and I knew that what I felt was more than friendship. We continued to talk regularly, as I still had two months left in Australia. I'd often get up at the crack of dawn or stay up until silly o'clock to talk to him. We'd known each other for four years, and all of a sudden something had shifted. One evening, he sent me an email inviting me to spend the weekend with him once I was back on UK soil. I said that I'd love to and he set to and booked everything. It was a total surprise and I had no idea where we were going or what was going to happen.

I met him at a train station, nearly sick with nerves and anticipation. But he was just the same Number 3 that I remembered. Silly and funny, but with this edge of the unpredictable. I couldn't quite work him out or pin him down and I loved that. It was so exciting to be with someone who wasn't afraid to take control and surprise me. As quite a confident, organised and adventurous person, I'd always been used to being the one that planned trips away and days out. Number 3 second guessed me and did it for me. Gold star to him.

We arrived at the most beautiful cottage in the Peak District. It was truly stunning. Here comes the bed rolling and squirty cream (unfortunately in that order) and although I clumsily ruined the possibility of sex for both of us, it was an amazing weekend, and one of many to come.

From my experience, relationships with long-term friends are very different to relationships with people that you have only connected with on a romantic basis. Although I was nervous, the whole thing felt oddly normal and natural. However, I seem to be a secret lover of long distance relationships, and as I went back to study in London for my final year of University, and Number 3 lived in Wales, we were to endure a five hour driving slog most weekends. Bloody hell, Em!

We made it work and… wait for it…. SEX HAPPENED! I'm feeling the virtual high fives right now, thanks. I'm so glad I waited for the right time and the right person. After several experiences of able-bodied male friends offering my first shag to me as they felt I 'deserved the experience', I'm glad I stuck to my guns and Number 3 was the guy. I won't go into too much detail but we have a great time, and being with someone that I can talk to and laugh with before, during and after sex is amazing. The fact that there's no pressure from either party, and we're both willing to try anything once, keeps things comfortable and exciting all at once. And that's what we're all looking for, right?

Almost three years later, I'm still mad about Number 3. We've also moved in together, which is everything I hoped it would be (although he's an untidy little sod…as they say, there's always room for improvement!). I now split my time between home and Rio De Janeiro, where I work as an accessibility consultant for the Olympic and Paralympic Games in 2016. See, I told you, secret love for long distance relationships that I can't seem to shift! Weirdly enough, I'm out in Rio at the moment and have just Skyped Number 3 and told him about my misfortunes in dating, during my teenage years. He just looked at me and smiled. 'Maybe it wasn't because of the chair, but because you're pretty….boisterous? Is boisterous the right word?' Although he's just practically likened me to a bulldog, I know what he means. 'Such a powerful personality…' he goes on, laughing, trying to redeem himself from the boisterous comment. But in all seriousness, maybe it's something worth thinking about. Many disabilities are undoubtedly obvious, as mine is. But just because it can be such a visual thing, we must not immediately assume that it automatically makes us less desirable.

Everyone has factors that either persuade or dissuade potential partners, and my wheelchair has not been a particular babe-magnet at times, but it has made me strong. I appreciate that that might be intimidating to some people, and if Number 3 and I did split, I'd definitely not be able to waltz into the nearest nightclub and pick up the next piece of eye-candy for a quickie. But, you know what? That's just fine with me. In short, I'm lucky. I'm lucky that the relationships, both romantic and platonic, that I've had in my 23 years have brought happiness, trust, and encouraged me to be the best possible version of myself. To round it all up, this quote always sticks in my head when I think about where I am now, and where I'd like to be: 'Love does not consist in gazing at each other, but in looking outward together in the same direction.' I hope I'll be looking in that same direction with Number 3 for years to come.

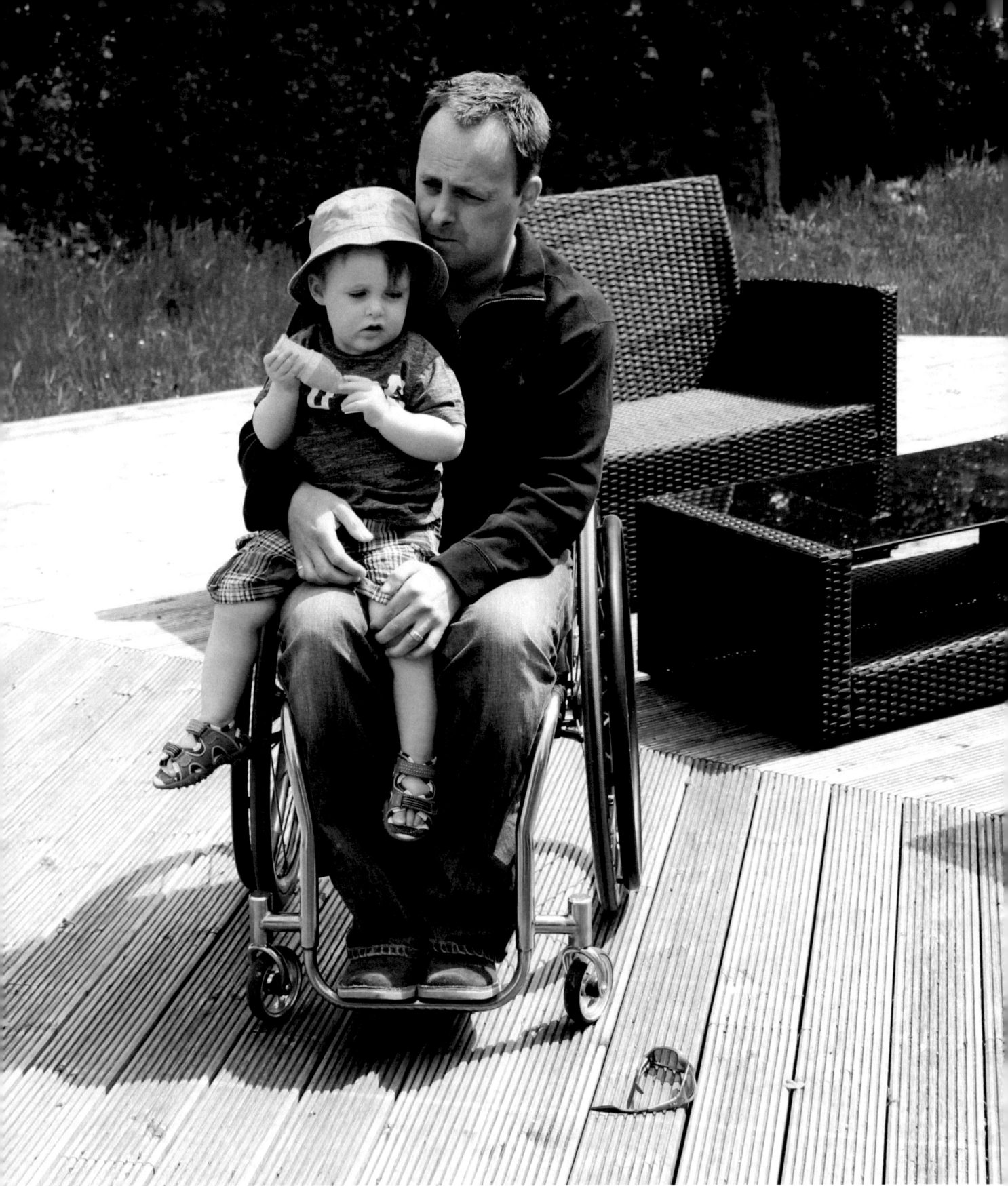

Ian Hosking was injured in 2004, has no movement or sensation from the chest down. and som
limitation in his hand function. Ian played wheelchair rugby for London Wheelchair Rugby
Club, one of the largest and most successful teams in Europe, for 8 years.

He has also given many talks about sport and injury to schools.

He now runs the Wheelchair Rugby Experience.

Ian's story

I've always loved cars and was a Mechanic running my own business. I was dropping a new car off to my mum, travelling along the M5 motorway, when a driver who had fallen asleep smashed me off the road. After rolling end over end a few times, the car ended up in a field, with its roof crushed - with me still in it. As it turns out, my neck was broken and I was to spend eleven months in hospital, two of which I would spend in a coma.

My whole life changed from that point, as I'm sure you can expect. I was in rehab for nine months, but only given the basic tools for living again. My relationship, job and independence were all to be put through great strain because of the incident, but more importantly all my focus and determination was taken up with learning how to look after myself, and even to wash and clean my teeth again, never mind worrying about life's big issues.

I can't really be angry toward the guy that knocked me off the road that day. He didn't intend to fall asleep, did he? Shit happens, it just happened to me that day, and I was left paralysed from the chest down, with some limitation to my hand function, with no stomach muscles and an inability to walk or even feel my legs.

Even though I'm the type of guy with the 'glass half full' mentality, it was tough avoiding the thoughts of 'Why me?', and not grieving for my previous life. But I kept telling myself that it could've been much worse. There could have been three outcomes that day. I could have died, become brain damaged, or been left paralysed. With paralysis, I got the best deal of the three, and I have to be grateful for that. In short, I had to 'man up'. My injury was never going to go away, so it was sink or swim time for me.

And that was the decider for me. Eighteen months after being in hospital, I found wheelchair rugby, and my life's turning point. All of a sudden, I was mixing with like-minded guys, some of whom had less function than me but could do more. This was a massive moment of clarity and determination.

Even though ball sports were never my thing, and I just used to race cars on race circuits, I was going to get fit and strong again and regain my confidence.

The day of the accident also massively changed my view on sex and relationships. My wife was also in the car, and broke her neck too. We were married for nine months at the time of the crash, and spent our first wedding anniversary in the hospital together. Possibly the first tetra couple in the world to ever do that! She'll always be the only person who was there at the time with me and went through it all beside me, but it wasn't fair on either of us to carry on the relationship. Two tetras aren't going to work – especially when she now needed 24 hour care due to her level of injury.

I'd say I had a straightforward, textbook sex life beforehand. Like a lot of men, I'd cum and go to sleep straight after! That's just nature playing tricks on us guys. At first, pushing to the pub in a wheelchair was scary, never mind talking to women! Rugby made me fitter and stronger, which made me more confident, but there was always the question in the back of my mind: 'What woman will want me now?' I don't think like that now, in fact I don't even consider myself disabled. My life is great; I'm just sat down! There's no woe about me, and I'm proud of that.

I've been married twice. Twelve or so months after leaving hospital, I started a new relationship and after around six years we got married. Unfortunately, it broke down. I'd changed as a person and became more focused on what I was looking for. It might've been maturity or how I changed after my injury, but I just knew I wanted something different. My injury made me realise that I had a second chance, and I didn't want to waste any of it. No longer would I plod on through life and take the easy option.

Equally, I was never one for playing any silly games, but I had learnt to make my own decisions and, to some extent, be selfish. My ex-wife is a great mother to our son, and didn't do anything wrong. I just knew I wasn't as happy as I could be, and recent life events had taught me that there's not enough time to allow those kinds of feelings to drag on.

For the next eight or so months, I tried internet dating. I enjoyed being able to tailor my settings to exactly what I was looking for. I'm really into feminine women, with their nails painted and hair and make-up done. I could filter my searches to help me find these women, and eventually I found someone. Of course, there were loads of women I contacted that I didn't receive any response from, and I knew it was likely to be the chair that put them off. But instead of worrying about it, I just figured that those kinds of people weren't for me. I needed someone who was willing to see past that. It took a few dates where no 'spark' was found, but there was never a stage where I thought 'I won't find anyone again'. I was confident I'd find someone who could overlook everything that had happened and see me.

A female physiologist once said to me, 'a man that can overcome spinal cord injury has to be made of strong stuff, and that's an attractive quality to a woman.' On one date, I got a massive 'spark' from a really cute girl. We got on so well, and the first date lasted nearly 24 hours! She was everything I had been looking for, but apparently I was not initially what she was looking for. She wanted a big six foot builder type who could sweep her off her feet… and I might struggle with that! However, she also wanted a 'doer' and someone who would look after her – and I'm definitely that. I'm the kind of person that, even if I can't physically do it, I'll make it happen. And that was that, and here we are, having the most amazing relationship and the best sex of our lives. I get on really well with her kids, plus mum and dad, too.

My son is nearly 4, and is happy to tell everyone, 'Daddy can't walk, but it doesn't matter.' The two of us together are quite a magnet for mums cooing – we frequently hear an 'awww!' when he's sat on my knee. He learnt, from a very young age, to balance himself on my knee and knew he'd fall off if he didn't. He was always motionless while I changed his nappy, and would never do that for his mum!

It isn't always plain sailing, though. When you have a spinal injury, people just naturally assume that you can't do anything. We once went away with my girlfriend's family, for example, and stayed in a hotel that didn't have any adapted rooms. Everyone was so concerned that I wouldn't be able to manage, but I got in and out of the bath quicker than it took her mum in the room next door! I've had my fair share of awkward moments, and anyone who has been to the National Spinal Injury Centre will know that there's a pile of dignity left at the front door. Well, mine is just part of the pile!

Most people that see someone in a wheelchair assume that it's just their legs that don't work. They have no idea I have no control over my bladder and bowels. The guy at the Ideal Home Show one year now knows, after I transferred onto a lovely bed he was selling and unfortunately emptied my bladder on it… I also had a 'spot of bother' one day: after I cleaned myself up quickly, I could still smell poo wherever I went all afternoon. I got home that evening to find that I still had poo on the back of my head from where I'd taken my t-shirt off. Lovely, a whole new meaning to the term shit-head!

It's not all embarrassing though, I have had some incredible opportunities that have come from the situation I would never have dreamed of! I'm great friends with the Captain of the 2012 Paralympic GB Wheelchair Rugby squad, and made it onto the GB Development Team myself. I didn't make it onto the full squad, partly because I probably wasn't good enough anyway, but also because having a sport as my full-time job isn't for me.

I've also done the London Marathon twice, but not without its 'situations'. Last time I did it, one other runner didn't see me and fell over the top of me! Three or four guys came to help me up, and ran with me for four or five miles until they couldn't keep up with me anymore! Yes, I use a wheelchair but I'm still fit, some people struggle to understand that.

I'm now having the best sex of my life and in a great place, but what do I miss about my sex life? I miss wanking, more than I miss walking! I can still get to wherever I want to in my chair, but I just can't do that anymore, and I thought I was pretty good at it…

If I wasn't on wheels myself now, I don't know if I'd have dated a girl in a chair before. But with what I know now and the experiences I've had, I would! In fact, maybe a wheelchair can be a positive thing, even a bonus. It breaks the ice, starts a conversation, and suddenly you're a bit different from the rest of them!

Isn't it amazing what life can throw at you after the most unexpected events?

The Love Lounge ♥

About

The Love Lounge is a safe online place, dedicated to every disabled person who wants to freely ask the questions we are sometimes too embarrassed to ask; somewhere to look for answers from people who have the experience of dating with a disability.

Dating with a disability can sometimes feel like a very isolating experience and we want to change that. The Love Lounge is here, because no one should be pushed out to the sidelines of life or left feeling lonely.

Our 'non-expert sexpert' panelists, Mik Scarlet and Emily Yates, are experienced, disabled, disability consultants who have had their share of dating highs and lows. Doctors, carers, and even our own families can feel very awkward talking about sex and disability so what better than to have somewhere to speak with people who know exactly what you are going through.

Drop your queries to us through our website, enhancetheuk.org or on socil media through Facebook Twitter.

Everybody wants to feel that they 'belong' and finding a sense of belonging with another person is very important to so many of us. Yet finding a 'soul mate,' for many people, is not so simple, especially when you have a disability.

Even if you're in an established relationship, all sorts of tensions and difficulties can crop up. It's especially hard if one of you becomes chronically sick, disabled or has an impairment, which changes.

It can then become, not only something you both need to get your head round, but could mean your partner now has to assist you in different ways and offer you 'care' in a way they haven't done before.

The dynamic of your relationship could change, sex might become physically or emotionally difficult, or you may end up feeling like you're living with your best friend, and sex is off the menu all together.

Maybe you're single and want to date, have fun, find the person of your dreams or even play the field a bit but are scared of ending up feeling like a novelty shag. Where do you look? How do you look? When do you mention an impairment or disability?

Living in a care home and maintaining or even establishing a relationship is no easy feat. Lack of information, attitudes, privacy, and access, are massive barriers. After all, how many double beds have you ever seen in a care home?

Questions and advice

"Should I brave using my prosthetic arm on the first date?"

"Hey guys, I have recently started internet dating since after Christmas and had a lot of interest on my profile, which is flattering! However, I only have one arm after losing it in a motorbiking accident in my teens. I usually only wear a shoulder prosthetic and skip my arm prosthetic as it can be a real pain – but should I brave it when going on the first few dates to avoid any awkwardness? What are your thoughts? Thanks x" - Michelle

Mik: "Hi Michelle,

I am a big fan of being up front, so I would go as you best feel comfortable. If you don't feel yourself when wearing your prosthetic then that might get in the way of the date. To me if anyone isn't keen on you because of your impairment then you've been saved from wasting time on a loser.

I had a mate at school that lost her arm at an early age and she never wore a prosthetic. She also never had any issues with guys. Her confidence was really attractive to us guys. Most of the men I know would much prefer someone who is happy with who they are than someone trying to be something they are not.

So I think my advice would be 'Be proud and leave the prosthetic at home.' Good luck and have a great time!"

"I'm 15 and the only wheelchair user in a mainstream school…"

"I'm 15 and the only wheelchair user in a mainstream school. I have a lot of friends but really like one guy in our group as more than that. He's nice to me but I don't think he looks at me in that way. How can I get him to notice me and not the

wheelchair?"
Rachel – Crawley

Hi Rachel, it's a great question, and a situation that many of us have been through. I think the one and only answer I can really give is 'be yourself, and let yourself shine. Most people are the best versions of themselves when they are relaxed and comfortable, so firstly work out what situations make you the most comfortable! It might be within a large group of friends, at a certain restaurant, or in the park opposite your house with a picnic and a book.

Whichever situation it might be, pluck up the courage to invite him along to things outside of school. This way you'll get to know each other on a more personal level. When you feel the time is right, arrange to do something with him that only involves you two: going for a coffee, to the cinema, taking him to one of your favourite places that is totally new to him etc. The more that you feel in control of the situation, the more confident you are likely to be. Hopefully you'll have loads of fun, and if he's still not making moves, maybe you could? At least you'll probably feel like you know him well enough to have 'the conversation' without it being awkward. Good luck!
Emily x

"I have Cerebral Palsy and can count my sexual experiences on the fingers of one hand."

"You invite people to share their stories of sexuality. I have cerebral palsy and can count my sexual experiences on the fingers of one hand. A psychiatrist once tried telling me this was because I was sexually deviant. I did not argue, but I felt he was mistaken and that he had no basis for advising me because he was not disabled and had not had any experience remotely related to disability. I would genuinely like to know how much you relate to this experience and its point of view. Thank you very much indeed." – James

Emily – "Hi James, many thanks for writing in. From one with CP to another, I can absolutely relate to your story. Seeing as 'deviant' really means 'differing from the norm'. We're probably all sexual deviants in our own ways, and this should in no way be seen as a negative thing. The problem is, the psychiatrist that you spoke to definitely displayed it negatively!

As I don't know the psychiatrist, I can't tell you whether he was capable of advising you or not, but what is coming through loud and clear is that fact that he seemed to give you little option to define, for yourself, what you sexually 'were' or 'were not'. And that's a problem that plagues society as a whole.

For example, society (in general) sees fewer sexual experiences as something to be ashamed of; society (in general) sees disability as an asexual concept, and these are the things that we are desperately trying to change.

In short, I sincerely hope that experiences like yours become fewer and more far between. Do write back in if you'd like any advice on any other aspect of disability, sex or relationships. Wishing you a lovely festive season, Emily x"

Mik – "Argh James, the old "you're deviant due to your disability" line eh? It is true that many non-disabled people seem to find the things that disabled people sometimes need to, or want to do, disconcerting. They like to say it is because they consider whatever fantasy or sexual predilection we admit to as being kinky, but I really think it is because they are uneasy with us wanting to not just have sex but enjoy it. Those in the medical and social professions can be the worst, as they really think they understand disabled people, as they have learned about us during their training. It takes a really skilled and rounded "expert" to be able to explore their own feelings around disability and sexuality, and to come out the other end being able to admit that we have all the same wants, dreams, desires and even fetishes as any non-disabled person might do. I would say never let anyone tell you that you are deviant, unless you are into some really weird shit.

I have had the exact same experience, just on a much more public scale. In the mid 90's I was a well-known TV presenter. I also sang in a rock band and we played on the fetish scene a lot. The Daily Mail ran a story "outing" me for being into kinky sex, yet only a year earlier the News Of The World ran a story with the headline of Wheelie Sexy, claiming they had found this new disabled sex symbol singer and presenter.

It seems is that if you appear sexual as a disabled person, that's fine, but if you actually have sex, and know what you might want out of sex, then that's just sick. It taught me that the wider public really do find the subject of disability and sex frightening and confusing, but then they are a repressed bunch mostly.

As well as being freaked out if disabled people express an interest in experimenting with sex, many people find the fact that we might need to try different stuff due to our specific physical needs equally troubling. I have written several articles on how many of the techniques used by disabled people, to enable them to have sex, would be of benefit to the wider non-disabled community but they are only ever featured in speciality magazines. The mainstream press find the whole idea of us teaching them something too bizarre to accept.

Without knowing what exactly it was that caused you to be called a deviant, all I can say is if you really are into fetishism or any other left field sexual activity, why not try visiting a local fetish club. It's one of the few places where people accept you as a sexual entity, and you might find someone that thinks what you are into is a perfect match for them.

I should also like to say that only being able to count your sexual partners on one hand is not a bad thing. I don't know how old you are but until I was nearly 30 I could have done the same with fingers to spare. Even today I could only use both hands and I was a famous TV presenter. It's not the quantity that matters, but the quality. I'd much rather have a few great nights to remember than a succession of crap shags."

"My daughter is 18 and has been blind from birth…"

"My daughter is 18 and has been blind from birth. She goes to college in our local area and is generally quite independent all round. My wife tells me that now she has started seeing a boy in her year at college. Part of me is happy, but a big part is being a protective father, especially because of her blindness. Should I just let her be a normal teenager?" - Tim

Mik: "Hi Tim, Arh the joys of fatherhood. Especially if you have daughters! It's all worry, worry, worry! But lets face it Tim, you'd be worried whether of not your daughter was visually impaired. It's your job, you're a dad!

I hope you know the answer to your question at heart. It's let her fly. She is an adult now, and is carving her place in the world. Part of that will be dating, no matter how much it hurts you inside. It's time to face up to the fact that your little girl is growing up, and be proud of how well she is doing.

This is a red-letter day really, and proof of how well you have raised her. She is obviously a confident, independent adult who is having no issues with getting out there and building a life for herself. Don't worry about her impairment, or what might happen with those pesky boys. Just support her, and wait to see if she needs a shoulder to cry on (if those aforementioned pesky boys do what teenage boys do, and act like fools).

Don't envy you though. I dread to think what I'd be like if I was a Dad!"

"I've just started seeing an amazing girl in the year above from school…"

I've just started seeing an amazing girl in the year above from school. She knows I'm partially blind and it's never been a big deal. But one of the only places we can hang out is at the cinema, which doesn't have many accessible movies with audio description. I don't want her to get bored with me! What other fun cheap dates could I take her on?" – Matthew, Liverpool

Hi! Some of my most memorable dates have been the cheapest! It's great that you want to mix it up a bit, and I'm sure she will love the date, whatever it is that you decide to do. I always think it's wonderfully interesting when you show somebody else 'your world', and introduce them to things that they've never experienced before. I play wheelchair basketball, and have taken my boyfriend to a game with me. He's able-bodied, and we've just started taking wheelchair ballroom dance classes! He loves it, as it's something that only I have been able to show him. Do you take part in any similar classes or clubs that you could introduce your girlfriend to? They're often free which is a huge plus! Failing that, going for a homemade picnic is always a winner! Or how about going back to basics and having a board game day at your house?! Totally free and SO MUCH FUN.

Emily x